HANDBOOK OF INTERNATIONAL FOOD REGULATORY TOXICOLOGY
Volume 1: Evaluations

HANDBOOK OF INTERNATIONAL FOOD REGULATORY TOXICOLOGY
Volume 1: Evaluations

Gaston Vettorazzi, M.D., Ph.D.
Scientist, Food Safety Program
World Health Organization, Geneva

and Professor of Experimental Toxicology
University of Milan

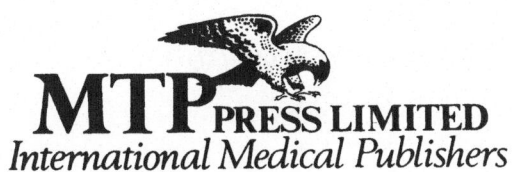

MTP PRESS LIMITED
International Medical Publishers

Published in the UK and Europe by
MTP Press Limited
Falcon House
Lancaster, England

Published in the US by
SPECTRUM PUBLICATIONS, INC.
175-20 Wexford Terrace
Jamaica, N.Y. 11432

ISBN-13: 978-94-011-7273-8   e-ISBN-13: 978-94-011-7271-4
DOI: 10.1007/978-94-011-7271-4

ACKNOWLEDGMENT

The author wishes to express his indebtedness to all the international experts in food additive toxicology, singly and collectively, who since 1956 have freely contributed their talent and time to the toxicological evaluation of pesticide chemicals within the context of the activities of the Joint FAO/WHO Expert Committee on Food Additives and other WHO Scientific Groups.

He also wishes to express his appreciation to those toxicologists and specialists, staff members of the Food and Agriculture Organization of the United Nations and the World Health Organization, who preceded him to his present responsibilities and cooperated in the development of the modern concept of toxicological evaluation and food additives at the international level.

Special acknowledgment and gratitude is given to Professor Rene Truhaut of the University of Paris, France and Member of the French Academy of Science for reviewing the manuscript and for encouraging the development of this work with his comments·

PREFACE

One of the striking features of our times is the increasing utilization of chemical products in different fields of human activities, as a result of the spectacular progress of chemical research. Our food supply has not been spared from this general trend, however, and chemical substances are being continuously incorporated in foodstuffs. Some of these substances are added to food for technological purposes such as preserving food from bacterial deterioration (antimicrobials), protecting it from oxidative changes (antioxidants), and improving its organoleptic characteristics (sweeteners, flavors, and flavor enhancers), or texture (stabilizers, emulsifiers, colorants). These substances are generally referred to as intentional food additives.

Chemical substances may also be found in food as a result of environmental or accidental contamination. Between these two categories of chemicals, a third class occupies an intermediate position, represented by chemical products utilized to control insect or fungus pests in agriculture and ectoparasites in animal husbandry. These products are currently referred to as pesticides and, due to some of their properties, such as chemical stability associated with scarce hydrosolubility, they may be found as residues in or on food from plant and animal origin. In addition, certain drugs that stimulate growth for accelerating productivity in animals may also be found as residues in edible animal tissues. These substances are referred to as unintentional food additives.

The utilization of additives in human food and animal feed brings about undeniable advantages for society. Similarly, the use of pesticides contributes to the preservation of our food resources and constitutes an important means in the fight against starvation.

However, consideration should be also given to the opposing viewpoint. It is an old notion, which Claude Bernard has repeatedly emphasized, that all chemical substances may evoke toxicological effects if the absorbed dose is sufficiently high and the time of exposure is sufficiently long. There are many examples demonstrating that very small doses which do not show any immediate apparent effect may cause harmful effects if the time of exposure extends over a lifetime of otherwise very long periods. They may cause serious symptoms of intoxication because of cumulative phenomena or they may elicit irreversible carcinogenic effects. The addition of chemical substances to food may thus establish optimal conditions for the manifestation of insidious forms of toxicity called long-term effects.

The possibility of causing long-term toxic effects by the use of food additives (food colors, antimicrobials, antioxidants, etc) has alerted toxicologists to require extensive and strict animal testing prior to utilization of these substances in food, in order to protect the health of the consumer.

In this regard, a pioneering role was played in the fifties at the international level by the European Committee of Chronic Toxicity (Eurotox). Around the same period, the International Union against Cancer was also active in evaluating the carcinogenic risk posed by chemical substances intentionally and unintentionally added to foodstuffs.

The World Health Organization (WHO) could not be indifferent to such an important problem and, since 1954, in collaboration with Food and Agriculture Organization of the United Nations (FAO), it has undertaken studies on the subject. An important decision was reached in September 1955, when a conference that met in Geneva, Switzerland, recommended that the Directors-General of the two organizations convene one or more expert committees, concerned with the technical and administrative aspects of the problem of chemical additives in food. The first meeting of a Joint FAO/WHO Expert Committee on Food Additives (JECFA) was held in Rome in December 1956, the most recent meeting (the 23rd) was held in Geneva in April 1979. A second committee, the Joint FAO/WHO Meeting on Pesticide Residues (JMPR) was initiated in 1963 and met annually thereafter; up to the present this committee held 15 sessions. The JMPR has been entrusted with the evaluation of the possible hazards to man arising from the occurrence of residues of pesticides in food.

After each session, these two committees prepare reports and monographs. The monographs contain summaries of technological, chemical, and toxicological studies which have been used to establish acceptable daily intakes (ADIs) and Maximum Residue Limits (MRLs). These publications have constituted the basis on which national regulatory agencies have formulated food laws for the protection of the consumer. Together with other reports dealing with toxicological methodology, these publications have considerably helped to establish the prestige of both FAO and WHO in the field of food safety.

The methodological approaches and the principles of interpretation of toxicological studies underwent continuous evaluation during the last three decades. In their reports, the JECFA and the JMPR have closely followed up the developments in this field and made recommendations. Unfortunately, their comments and suggestions are scattered over many publications and a systematic assemblage of the major conclusions will certainly facilitate the interested parties to locate significant information.

Dr. Gaston Vettorazzi, a WHO staff member since 1972, who actively participated in the deliberations of both the JECFA and JMPR has undertaken, with the present volume, a systematic collection of toxicological methodology and principles of interpretation of experimental findings. I am pleased to write the foreword to this book, since I have been connected with the activities of these two international committees since their outset.

In the last paragraph of his introduction, the author expressed the hope that his work would be of help to all those engaged in research and work in the field of food additives, food contaminants, and pesticides.

I don't think I am biased by my friendship with him when I say that his hope is sure to be fulfilled. He has succeeded in the task he set himself to do. His book meets a real international need and should occupy a place of honor in the book-shelves not only of toxicologists, but also in that of medical doctors, food hygienists, food technologists, agronomists, administrators, food regulatory personnel, as well as industrialists and consumer advocates.

Professor Rene Truhaut
Professor of Toxicology
Member of the "Institut de France"
(Academy of Science)

Contents

INTRODUCTION

The increase in the number of chemical substances used or proposed for use in or on food has imposed upon public health departments and other governmental agencies the responsibility for deciding
whether a certain substance should be permitted to be used by food
processors. This matter was stressed several years ago by national
and international organizations among which should be mentioned the
European Committee of Chronic Toxicity (EUROTOX), the International
Union Against Cancer (UICC), the National Academy of Science (NAS),
the Food and Agriculture Organization of the United Nations (FAO) and
the World Health Organization (WHO).

To limit consideration to the last two organizations, in 1953 the
Sixth World Health Assembly (the organ that determines the policies
of WHO) expressed the view that the increasing use of various chemical
substances by the food industry had in the last few decades created a
new public health problem which might usefully be investigated (1).
The same problem was subsequently examined in 1954 by the WHO
Executive Board (the organ that gives effect to the decisions and policies of the World Health Assembly), and it was recommended that
WHO, in cooperation with FAO, should collect and disseminate information on selected groups of chemical additives used in food, including testing techniques and relevant legislation (2).

The Council of FAO, at its Twentieth Session in 1954, also recognized that the problem of food additives was of growing importance
with respect both to motivation and food production and distribution,
and it requested the Director-General of FAO to consider the kind of
work which FAO could appropriately undertake in the field of food additives, in association with the World Health Organization, taking into
account any recommendations made by the Joint FAO/WHO Expert
Committee on Nutrition (3).

1

At the fourth session of this above committee, the desirability of a uniform approach to this problem was discussed. Attention was drawn to the 1) wide divergences in the legislative measures adopted, or proposed for adoption, in different countries; 2) conflicting evidence relating to individual food additives and the differences in interpreting this evidence; and 3) serious lack of data regarding many food additives with regard to both their purity and to the health hazards involved in their use. It was felt that the groups which had been independently concerned with this subject were not only limited in membership, but that their activities in virtually identical fields have already led to undesirable duplication of effort, and might, without adequate coordination, result in conflicting recommendations. The desirability of calling a conference of representatives of the existing groups working on this subject, together with appropriate representatives of member nations as might be interested and would be prepared to send delegates, was suggested (4).

This conference met in Geneva, Switzerland in 1955 and recommended to the Directors-General of WHO and FAO to convene one or more expert committee to be concerned with the technical and administrative aspects of the problem of chemical additives in food, namely: 1) to formulate general principles governing the use of food additives, with special reference to their legal authorization, based on appropriate consideration of their harmlessness, standards of purity, limits of tolerance, and the social, economic, psychological, and technological reasons for their use taking into account the work already done in this field by national and international bodies; 2) to recommend, as far as practicable, suitable uniform methods for the physical, chemical, biochemical, pharmacological, toxicological, and biological examination of food additives and of any breakdown products formed from them during processing, for the pathological examination of experimental animals, and for the assessment and interpretation of the results. This conference defined food additives as non-nutritive substances which are added intentionally to food, generally in small quantities to improve its appearance, flavor, texture or storage properties (5).

Similarly, following a recommendation of the European Commission in Agriculture at its tenth session in 1958, the Food and Agriculture Organization of the United Nations convened in 1959 a panel of experts on the use of pesticides in agriculture (6). This panel reviewed some major problems on the use of pesticides, such as the role of pesticides in agriculture, their efficient and safe use, and the potential risks to useful insects, livestock, and domestic animals as well as to consumers of foodstuffs, and touched on the legislative control of pesticide residues. Noting that questions related to intentional food additives used by the food processing industry were already being dealt with by another expert committee, the panel recommended that studies be undertaken jointly by FAO and WHO on: 1) the hazards to consumers arising from pesticide residues in and on food and feedstuffs; 2) the establishment of principles governing the setting up pesticide tolerances; 3) the feasibility of preparing an international code for toxicological and residue data required in achieving the safe use of pesticides;

and 4) the ways and means of disseminating to the public adequate information on precautionary measures employed to protect consumer interests. In order to implement these recommendations, a joint meeting between a WHO expert committee on pesticide residues and an FAO panel of experts met in Rome in 1961 (7). At this meeting, problems were examined and guidelines laid down relating to the control of the use of pesticides, toxicological investigations required, and basic requirements for the establishment of residue tolerances and scientific and regulatory information services. In particular, it was recommended that studies be undertaken to evaluate the evidence, including both published and unpublished toxicological and other pertinent data, on those pesticides known to leave residues in food when used according to good agricultural practice, and that conclusions be issued in the form of acceptable daily intakes (ADIs) for man supported by explanations of the basis for each value.

In 1962 an FAO conference on pesticides in agriculture (8) was held in Rome and was attended by national delegates. Its primary purpose was to formulate and recommend a plan for future action concerning scientific, legislative, and regulatory aspects of the use of pesticides in agriculture. The conference noted that there were no published ADI figures for man and that such figures would be of great assistance to countries that were able to establish pesticide tolerances in food.

In May 1963 the Sixteenth World Health Assembly approved the establishment of a joint FAO/WHO program on food standards with the Codex Alimentarius Commission as its principal organ. Within the framework of this program, a Codex Committee on Pesticide Residues was set up by the Commission in June of the same year (10). The second FAO/WHO joint conference on food additives (11) which was held during the same month, noted that pesticide residues had been dealt with in separate program. In September-October 1963, the WHO Expert Committee on Pesticide Residues and the FAO Committee on Agriculture met jointly in Geneva, Switzerland (12) and in 1965 in Rome, Italy (13). These meetings were concerned with establishing acceptable daily intakes for man. The reports from these meetings and the supporting documents were then considered by the FAO Working Party on Pesticide Residues with the view to recommending tolerances and appropriate methods of analysis (14).

The first meeting of the Joint FAO/WHO Expert Committee on Food Additives was held in Rome in 1956, and the most recent (the 23rd) was held in Geneva in April 1979. Similarly, the Joint Meetings of the WHO Expert Committee on Pesticide Residues and the FAO groups of experts on pesticide residues have been held annually since 1966, the most recent being held in Geneva in December 1979.

During the 23 years of activities of the committee on food additives and the 15 years of action of the committee on pesticide residues, many publications have been issued by the two sponsoring organizations on this subject. These publications contain the deliberations/recommendations of these expert groups as well as summaries of toxicological data, specifications for identity and purity, recommended toxicological testing procedures, and principles of interpretation of experimental findings.

Acceptable daily intake figures (ADIs) for the most commonly used food additives and ADI figures and recommended maximum residue limits (MRL) for a variety of pesticide chemicals are also included.

Comments and recommendations regarding testing procedures and principles of interpretation of experimental findings are widely distributed throughout many documents and no single volume is available condensing in a systematic form all the pertinent material. Since one may, consequently, find it difficult to locate the relevant information, this book was designed to permit an easy access to it.

It should, however, be noted that some of the extracted statements regarding views on testing procedures might reflect opinions which may no longer be tenable today. In spite of this, they have been equally recorded and referenced in order to offer the reader a useful historical background to better appreciate current positions.

Finally, it should be borne in mind that the book supplies only a systematic presentation and by no means a critical review of the material quoted.

It is hoped that this work will be valuable to individuals or groups involved in the toxicological assessment of food additives and pesticide chemicals.

REFERENCES

1. World Health Organization, Resolution WHA, 6. 16. Off. Rec. Wld Hlth Org. 48. 22, 1953.
2. World Health Organization, Resolution EB13. R47. Off. Rec. Wld Hlth Org. 52. 20, 1954.
3. Food and Agriculture Organization, Report of the Council of FAO, twentieth session, 27 September - 8 October 1954. Rome, Resolution No. 4/20, 1954.
4. World Health Organization, Fourth report of the Joint FAO/WHO Expert Committee on Nutrition. FAO Nutrition Meetings Report Series, No. 9; Wld Hlth Org. Techn. Rep. Ser. , No. 97, 1955.
5. World Health Organization, Joint FAO/WHO Conference on Food Additives. FAO Nutrition Meetings Report Series, No. 11; Wld Hlth Org. techn. Rep. Ser. , No. 107, 1956.
6. FAO, Report of the FAO Panel of Experts on the Use of Pesticides in Agriculture. Meeting Report No. 1959/3 (mimeographed document No. FAO/59/6/4357), 1959.
7. WHO/FAO, Principles governing consumer safety in relation to pesticide residues. Report of a WHO Expert Committee on Pesticide Residues held jointly with the FAO Panel of Experts on the Use of Pesticides in Agriculture. FAO Plant Production and Protection Division Report No. PL/1961/11; Wld Hlth Org. techn. Rep. Ser. , 240, 1962.
8. FAO, Report of the FAO Conference on Pesticides in Agriculture. Meeting Report No. PL/1962/17, 1962.
9. World Health Organization, Handbook of Resolutions and Decisions, Vol. 1, p. 157, 1973.
10. Joint FAO/WHO Codex Alimentarius Commission. Report of the first Session. Alinorm 63/12, p. 11, 1963.

11. WHO/FAO, Second Joint FAO/WHO Conference on Food Additives. FAO Nutrition Meetings Report Series, No. 34; Wld Hlth Org. techn. Rep. Ser. , No. 264, 1963.
12. WHO/FAO, Evaluation of the toxicity of pesticide residues in food. FAO Nutrition Meetings Report Series, No. PL/1963/13; WHO/ Food Add./23, 1964.
13. WHO/FAO, Evaluation of the toxicity of pesticide residues in food. FAO Meeting Report, No. PL/1965/10; WHO/Food Add./26. 65, 1965.
14. FAO, Report of the Second Session of the FAO Working Party on pesticide residues. FAO Meeting Report, No. PL/1965/12, 1965.

Chapter 1

General Principles in the Toxicological Evaluation of Food Additives

1. INTRODUCTION

Since the outset of their activities in the field of safety evaluation of food additives, the WHO/FAO Expert Committee on Food Additives and other expert groups in the World Health Organization have dealt with the general principles in the toxicological evaluation of chemicals added to food either specifically in special meetings (1,2,3) or occasionally during the course of their meetings aimed at formulating toxicological decisions regarding these substances. This chapter aims at bringing together the most important observations, remarks or suggestions concerning general principles of toxicological evaluation, procedures for testing and methodological approaches made by these international expert bodies since 1956.

There are reasons why activities on the safety evaluation of food additives have been carried out at the international level. In effect, one of the major problems in connection with food additives is the satisfactory control of their use. In many countries special agencies or departments are responsible for such control and in some, supporting scientific facilities are available. In many others, however, there is no adequate machinery by which those responsible for public health can usefully handle these problems. Furthermore, the solutions that may be effective in one country are not necessarily applicable to another, since the nature of foods consumed, pattern of the local diet, and environmental conditions of life vary greatly. It was therefore recommended (4) that FAO and WHO should carry out a survey of the literature dealing with the biological properties of the more important chemical substances that might be proposed for use as food additives and submit this information to an expert committee for evaluation (5).

A joint FAO/WHO program was therefore initiated with the object of making systematic evaluations of food additives and providing advice

7

to member states of FAO and WHO on the control of these chemicals
and on related health aspects. The hope was expressed that this advice
will also help to render the legislation of countries more uniform with
regard to the control of food additives and thus facilitate international
trade. The two bodies responsible for implementing the program are
the Joint FAO/WHO Expert Committee on Food Additives and the Committee on Food Additives of the Joint FAO/WHO Codex Alimentarius
Commission. The respective functions of these two bodies are indicated below.

The Joint FAO/WHO Expert Committee on Food Additives in an
expert body composed of members invited by FAO and WHO and who
serve in their individual capacity as scientists and not as representatives of their governments. The main terms of reference of this expert
committee are to establish specifications for identity and purity for
food additives and to evaluate the toxicological data and recommend,
where possible, acceptable daily intakes for man (ADIs). This expert
committee also acts in an advisory capacity to the Codex Committee on
Food Additives, a committee which is attended by representatives of
member governments. Through the Codex Alimentarius Commission
it proposes levels for additives in various foods to governments for
international acceptance.

The substances to be considered at a meeting at the expert committee are often selected by the Codex committee. In making this selection priorities are given to those substances used extensively in food
entering international trade in substantial amounts. However, substances used extensively in domestic food in individual countries are
also considered by the expert committee upon request from governmental authorities. The fact that a substance has not yet been considered by the expert committee does not necessarily imply any doubt
about its technical usefulness or safety in use.

Before each meeting, every effort is made by the WHO and FAO
secretariat to collect as many relevant published and unpublished data
as possible on toxicology and specifications for identity and purity of
the substance to be examined. After each meeting a report is issued
which contains a description of the general principles used in the evaluation as well as a brief summary of the deliberations on the substances
listed on the agenda. Following each meeting, one or more documents
are published in addition to the report mentioned above (6).

Several hundred food additives have been examined and about 50
publications have been issued by the two sponsoring organizations on
this subject. These publications contain deliberations and recommendations as well as summaries of toxicological studies with respective
references and chemical specifications for identity and purity for the
most commonly used food additives.

In its 23 years of existence this committee has reviewed the most
important of the intentional food additives that are used widely and in
significant quantities for improving the storage and processing of food.
In addition to evaluating specific substances the committee and two
working groups (2,3) have played an important role in encouraging the
development of toxicity testing and in outlining procedures for the
evaluation of the results of toxicological studies in terms of the safety

in use of food additives When its terms of reference were expanded, the committee also dealt with some of the most important of the food contaminants that were known to be hazardous to health, notably the heavy metals mercury, lead and cadmium. At its successive meetings, the committee has responded promptly and sensitively to new biological discoveries that appeared to have a bearing on the safety aspects of food additives and contaminants.

There are, however, a large number of chemicals in food that have never been examined. Some of these are intentional additives, the most important and largest group being flavoring substances of which only a few have been evaluated. Only a few of the adventitious additives such as residues of processing aids, residues of animal feed additives and substances migrating from packaging materials into food have been evaluated. Furthermore, comparatively little detailed attention has been paid to the many contaminants with known or suspected toxicity, or to natural constituents of foods that have a toxic potential.

The problem raised by the large numbers of food additives and contaminants that have not yet been evaluated was recognized earlier (234) and a recommendation was made that WHO should consider ways and means to expedite the FAO/WHO program on food additives. Subsequently, the World Health Assembly adopted a resolution (WHA 30.47) concerning the evaluation of the health effects of chemicals generally, and requested the Director-General to undertake a study on the long-term strategies and the possible options for international cooperation in this field. As a first step in the study, a consultation on the implementation of resolution WHA 30.47 was held in Geneva in September 1977 and the possible tasks to be undertaken were identified and a number of options for their implementation were proposed.

This progress was noted with satisfaction and it was recommended that in any option adopted following the study recommended in WHA 30.47, food additives and contaminants should be considered as one of the priority group of substances for accelerated and systematic evaluation. Many of the compounds already tested and evaluated related to food could serve as models for assessing the validity of testing methods and the appropriateness of procedures for evaluation of the effects on health of chemicals generally.

In considering the problem of the number of compounds, it was recognized that it would be impossible to undertake within a reasonable period of time full toxicological studies with all the known food additives and contaminants.) Furthermore, the carrying out of such studies would represent an unjustifiable expenditure of effort, assigning equal importance to substances posing unequal risks without contributing significantly to the protection of public health. It is thus necessary to set priorities for testing and evaluation of these substances. The mechanism for setting these priorities was discussed extensively and it was stressed that the assignment of a priority is not a substitute for a proper evaluation, but merely a means to assure that the compounds with the greatest toxic potential are studied first in preference to those with a lower priority.

The assessment of priorities is based on various types of information:

a. Structure-activity relationships in as much as they serve to predict potential toxicity;
b. Human exposure, in terms of the range of food containing the substance, its concentration, and its intake in the diet;
c. Available toxicological data;
d. Prior experience of human use;
e. Metabolic fate in animals and man;
f. Use in special populations at risk such as pregnant women, the very young and those with special disabilities.

Using the above criteria, compounds can be classified into various categories. Substances with the lowest priority for testing and evaluation are those that by their structural characteristics are considered to be innocuous and are consumed in very low quantities. Compounds with high priority have structural features either known to be associated with toxicity or are of unknown toxic potential and are present in human food in appreciable quantities.

Most of the compounds are expected to fall somewhere between the two extremes, and their priority for testing and evaluation should be set accordingly.

A new proposal was noted which provides a useful procedure for the estimation of the toxic potential of chemicals from various structural features (235). It was observed that this method as well as other procedures for estimating toxic potential from structure-activity relationships should be explored.

Furthermore, the need was recognized to establish as a matter of urgency an inventory of intentional and unintentional food additives that have not yet been evaluated, and recommended that an interdisciplinary working group of experts be convened by FAO/WHO to establish this inventory. The compounds in the list should then be classified by these experts in terms of potential toxicity and extent of use to establish priorities for testing and evaluation, and a number of high priority compounds should be selected for future evaluation (236).

It was recommended that compounds with very high priorities set according with the criteria outlined above should be subjected to a comprehensive animal toxicity testing program as recommended in previous reports. Compounds with lower priorities, that is those considered innocuous from a chemical point of view and consumed in very small quantities, will not necessarily require as comprehensive testing as the high priority substances. The precise tests to be used for the low priority compounds were not recommended but it was indicated that WHO should explore the means to assemble a working group of experts who would evaluate available testing procedures and would issue guidelines for an abbreviated testing program. It is, furthermore, understood that a compound may be reclassified into a higher priority class in the light of results obtained from such a toxicological screening. It would then have to be studied more extensively (236).

2. PRINCIPLES GOVERNING THE
USE OF FOOD ADDITIVES

The need and importance of food additives have been stressed on several occasions. The increase in the number of chemicals used or proposed for use in or on food has imposed upon public health authorities and other governmental agencies the responsibility for deciding whether or not such substances should be employed. The socio-economic position of a country is an important factor in arriving at such decision. Additives can contribute greatly to the preservation of food; for example, they can help prevent the wastage of seasonal surpluses. In economically underdeveloped countries, lack of modern storage facilities and the inadequacy of transport and communications may increase the necessity of using certain food additives for purposes of food preservation. In tropical regions, where high temperature or humidity favor microbial attack and increase the rate of development of oxidative rancidity, a wider use of antimicrobial agents and antioxidants may be justified than in more temperate climates. In these regions possible risks associated with the increased use of food additives must be weighed against the benefits in the form of preventing wastage and making more food available in areas in which it is needed. In these circumstances, however, food additives should be used to supplement the effectiveness of traditional methods of food preservation rather than to replace these methods.

In countries which are technically and economically highly developed, the availability of adequate facilities for refrigerated transport and storage reduces, even if it does not eliminate, the need for antimicrobial agents. In these countries, however, there is an increasing demand for more attractive foods, for uniformity of quality and for a wide choice of foods at all seasons of the year. Large quantities of many of the foods consumed have to be transported from distant producing areas, a fact which may create special transport and storage problems. For such purposes the variety of useful food additives is great and their employment promotes the better utilization of the available foods.

The extent to which food additives are likely to be needed and their nature will therefore vary considerably from region to region and even from country to country. In decisions concerning the use of an additive, attention should be given to its technological usefulness, protection of the consumer against deception, the use of inferior techniques in processing and, above all, to the evidence bearing on the safety for use of the substance (7).

The same concept has been more recently reiterated in connection with the food-population equation. In fact the continuing increase in the world population without a comparable increase in the available amount of conventional foodstuffs must stimulate further efforts to develop new sources of food. In addition to ensuring the safety of these new foods, there is also a need to ensure their palatability and acceptability to consumers, and food additives will thus be required for the purposes of preserving, texturizing, flavouring, and colouring them. Therefore, the work of this committee can be looked upon as a means of ensuring wholesome nutritious foods for the present and future generations (8).

Food additives should be used only after authorization by the appropriate authorities and their legal control should be based on the system of permitted or positive lists. Two factors have to be taken into account in evaluating a substance proposed for use as a food additive, namely technological efficacy and safety in use. The criteria for both must be satisfied before a substance can be formally accepted as a food additive (9).

There are a number of circumstances in which there is technological justification for the use of acceptable food additives to the advantage of the consumer. The most important are: (a) maintaining the nutritional quality of the food, (b) enhancing the keeping quality or stability with resulting reduction in food wastage, (c) making food attractive to the consumer, and (d) providing essential aids in food processing (10). However, there are situations in which food additives should not be used. Apart from questions of toxicity there are a number of circumstances in which the use of certain food additives is not in the best interest of the consumer and, therefore, should not be permitted. The most important are : (a) to disguise the use of faulty processing and handling techniques, (b) to deceive the consumer, (c) to reduce the nutritive value of a food substantially, and (d) good manufacturing practices which are economically feasible (11). In conclusion, the use of a food additive should be technologically justified on the basis of advantage to the community and the consumer, and the level of use should not exceed the lowest level that is effective in good manufacturing practice (12,13).

The most important factor for the acceptance of a substance as a food additive is the establishment of its safety in use. This implies that an adequate toxicological evaluation has to be made (13). This principle was clearly stressed in the committee's first report. While it is impossible to establish absolute proof of the nontoxicity of a specified use of an additive for all human beings under all conditions, critically designed animal tests of the physiological, pharmacological and biochemical behavior of a proposed additive can provide a reasonable basis for evaluating the safety of use of a food additive at a specified level of intake. However, it has been stressed that the principle for any decision to use an intentional additive must be based on the considered judgment of properly qualified scientists that the intake of the additive will be substantially below any level which could be harmful to consumers. The decision as to a safe level should be based on knowledge of the maximum dietary level that produces no unfavorable response in test animals, of the severity and type of response in animals above that level, and of the estimated potential intake of the additive.

Toxicological considerations should include not only the food additive as such, but also substances produced in the food by the action of the additive and the possibility of the formation of toxic substances from the additive during processing, storage and household preparation. The possible interaction of additives should also be borne in mind.

In addition, attention should be given to the question of whether the combined effects of a number of additives with similar toxicological properties might produce an undesirable summation of reactions. There may be substances which, because of some special biological property, may have the effect of making other additives harmful. Evidence bearing on these points deserves consideration in decisions pertaining to the use of additives.

Judgment as to safety must recognize that there may be groups within a population which, because of physiological state or organic disease, may be specially sensitive to the additive concerned. These groups include those suffering from a variety of chronic diseases; for example, malnutrition, parasitosis and certain degenerative conditions. In this connection, it must be emphasized that while easily identifiable foods are readily avoided, this is not so with some food additives.

It is therefore clear that the study and laboratory testing of a substance, and the scientific advice given concerning its use, may well differ from country to country.

Permitted additives should be subjected to continuing observation for possible deleterious effects under changing conditions of use. They should be reappraised whenever indicated by advances in knowledge. Special recognition in such reappraisals should be given to improvements in toxicological methodology. In some countries additives are employed without the safeguard provided by appropriate study. The limited facilities for toxicological work in many countries should be expanded in order to meet the needs for these investigations. There should likewise be a continuing increase in the international cooperation and exchange of information in this area (14).

The committee has frequently reiterated the general principles laid down in its first report concerning the safe use of food additives. However, it should be pointed out that the absolute safety of the foods themselves cannot be guaranteed since natural components of normal foods may exhibit toxic properties. By contrast, the scrutiny to which food additives are subjected in arriving at a toxicological evaluation makes for their safety in practice. The potential hazard, if any, that the use of a food additive may present to the consumer must be weighed against the benefits that it confers; for example, a food additive may provide protection against the development in food of microbial toxins or mycotoxins.

When several additives are used in a food, the most important factor to be considered is the level of exposure of the consumer to each food additive rather than the total number used. In fact, the use of a number of food additives to achieve a technological effect, each at a lower level than would be needed if it were used alone, may provide an additional measure of safety, as long as there are no undesirable interactions between them. Such interactions may be chemical or biological in nature. Considerations should be given to possible chemical interactions between food additives that might yield toxic substances, thus precluding the simultaneous use of the additives in the same food. In regarding biological interactions, it has been acknowledged that there is the theoretical possibility of some subtle potentiation of toxicity, but in practice such an effect has rarely been encountered. Compounds that are closely related in chemical structure or function may exhibit additive and, more rarely, synergistic biological effects. In several instances acceptable daily intake figures have been allocated to groups of such compounds, thus providing a safeguard in the event of a number of such food additives being used in a single food.

In the years that have elapsed since the publication of the first committee report, the importance of the general principles concerning the safe use of food additives has been repeatedly stressed. It has been also emphasized that, provided these principles are adhered to, the goal of the safety in use of food additives is attainable in practice (15).

Recently attention was called to the importance of information on food additives and food contaminants to developing and developed countries. Insisting on the aspect of world-wide population growth and rises in standards of living which constantly call for increased food supply, it was observed that increased food production as well as better protection and preservation of food supplies and use of better processing techniques in line with advances in food technology imply an increased use of food additives. Furthermore, increasing industrialization, which may lead to contamination of the environment and hence of food, calls for vigilance to prevent health hazards from such contaminants. In an effort to increase supplies, new food sources are being developed. The safety of such food should be given close attention.

It was recognized that the gorwing concern in industrialized countries about carcinogenic, mutagenic and teratogenic contaminants is shared by many developing countries, as is also the concern about special hazards faced by vulnerable population groups; and that cooperation of scientists familiar with the circumstances and needs of developing countries could materially assist the international work on food contaminants and additives, particularly to help in recognizing and avoiding any pitfalls relating to conditions in their countries and to facilitate their utilizing the results of the committee's work (16).

Information on food additives should not be limited to supply the scientific basis for legislation or regulation, but should reach the users. In this respect it has been agreed that in principle, consumers should be informed of the presence of additives in their food. Label declaration is the most effective method of achieving this result, but in some countries alternative approaches have been adopted. Thus, for example in the United States, standards of identity for foods have been established which are available to the public and which list the permissive ingredients. These standards require the label declaration of only certain specified classes of additives. Provided that strict legal control over the use of additives is exercised, label declaration is necessary to inform the consumer rather than to protect his health.

Exceptions may have to be made for certain classes of food. For example, some foods are normally sold in an unpackaged form and in such circumstances label declaration becomes impractical. In other instances, the addition of certain additives is sufficiently evident and therefore lebel declaration may not be necessary.

Since most consumers are uninformed as to the nature and purposes of additives, confusion and suspicion tend to be created in their minds if the manufacturer is compelled by law to declare the chemical name and concentration of the additive which is used. Therefore, simple declarations of the presence of a particular class of additives such as "artificial color added" or "artificial flavor added" are sufficient.

When non-nutritive additives are deliberately employed to replace nutrients in the preparation of foods for special uses, it is clearly necessary to identify the use for which the food is intended in order to avoid deception of the consumer (17).

In developing criteria for food additive control, it has been observed that factors other than toxicology should be taken into account. For instance, when a new food additive is proposed for use, clear evidence must be available to show that benefits to the consumer will ensue. In classes of foods which constitute a considerable proportion of the diet, the use of intentional additives should, in principle, be limited. The presence of harmful impurities in food additives can be excluded most effectively by the establishment of specifications of purity (18).

However, a word of caution was expressed on premature replacement of suspect chemicals by less tested substances. In effect, sometimes the results of a toxicological test on a widely used material are difficult to interpret and this may lead to some uncertainty about its safety. A general problem will arise in relation to food if a long used and well tested material is found to have some manifestation of toxicity which is difficult to intepret and consequently is replaced by a substance which is untested or less well tested. The problem may be examplified by the replacement of trichloroethylene by methylene chloride. There are similar kinds of examples with industrial chemicals and pesticides as well (19).

A special problem is represented by the use of food additives in baby foods or any food that is directly or by implication represented as being intended for feeding to infants and young children. A distinction between baby food suitable for infants up to the age of 12 weeks and those designed to be given to the older infant has been made. On developmental ground this is an arbitrary distinction. However, it is likely that the detoxicating mechanisms, the permeability of certain tissues, and other protective mechanisms of infants aged up to 12 weeks may not have developed to a point where they are able to cope with substances that present no problem to the adult. There is little evidence regarding the age of maturation of detoxicating mechanisms, particularly regarding individual variability. It may be assumed that by the end of the twelfth week most of the necessary protective mechanisms have developed. Few additives have been investigated in relation to their effects on very young children. It is therefore prudent that foods intended for infants under 12 weeks old should contain no additives at all. Such food would include infant formulas (and other milk-based preparations), cereal-based baby foods, and "strained" foods and fruit juices. Certain cereal-based baby foods, "strained" foods, and "junior" foods that are intended for older babies may contain additives and should be adequately labelled to ensure that they are not consumed by infants under 12 weeks.

The availability of "junior" and "strained" foods confers an advantage in that the infant may be given a diet more varied and therefore often nutritionally more satisfactory than it would otherwise receive.

Although after 12 weeks detoxicating and other protective mechanisms may be adequately developed, it must be remembered that, in terms of caloric intake per kilogram of body weight, young children consume up to three times as much as adults. This factor needs to be borne in mind when considering levels of additives in foods designed for young children.

Additives designed for inclusion in baby foods, particularly those for infants under 12 weeks of age, should be submitted to more extensive toxicological investigations including evidence of safety in young animals and technological justifications should be given less weight than in the case of foods intended for older babies or adults.

Finally, concern was expressed that in addition to food specifically intended for adults may be eaten by children; in particular, processed dairy products, bread, and biscuits, all of which may contain additives, are often fed to babies instead of cereal-based foods specifically prepared for infants and the attention of appropriate public health and other expert bodies should be drawn to this problem (20).

3. CONSIDERATIONS ON THE PHYSICAL AND CHEMICAL IDENTIFICATION OF FOOD ADDITIVES

The need for and value of specifications for identity and purity of food additives have been emphasized on several occasions (21-23).

It is necessary that food additives, many of which are not single chemical substances, should be identifiable in chemical and physical terms. The components of such mixtures should be described and the limits of reproducible composition defined. Such identification is essential in order to compare the results of toxicity testing and to ensure that the additive tested is the additive which is used in practice (24).

This aspect has been elaborated in considerable detail emphasizing the need for establishing specifications for the identity and purity of food additives at an international level. It was noted that for many years national pharmacopoeias and similar compendiums have contained specifications for the more important drugs and drug components, and that the International Pharmacopoeia published by WHO has provided similar data on the international level. In recent years, certain governments have begun to prepare specifications for the chemicals that enter the national food supply. However, there is a great need to prepare such data on an international level (25, 26).

The value of specifications can be summarized in the following ways:

Value in protecting the consumer. Whereas a natural food may vary in composition, sometimes to a considerable degree in undefined ways, considerations of public health dictate that, as a matter of principle, additives to food should be of known composition and purity. In fact, modern methods make it possible to produce chemicals of greater purity and uniformity of synthesis than is usually achieved by derivation from substances of natural origin. The adoption of official specifications for food additives would give assurance to the consuming public that substances meeting established standards of purity are available for use in food (25, 27, 28).

Value for regulatory purposes. At the present time most food legislation merely indicates by name the substances which may be used in a particular food. It is a well-known fact that chemicals are produced in a variety of technical and refined grades. Toxicological evaluation, which is a costly and time-consuming procedure, must be related to the particular grade or quality of chemical intended for use in food. The adoption of specifications for purity for food additives would provide a means of accurate identification of the additive for regulatory purposes and would limit the known undesirable ingredients or contaminants to acceptable tolerance levels (29-31).

Value to industry. The existence of specifications, agreed upon by qualified specialists, serves to ensure a degree of reproducibility and of conformity to criteria of quality which are acceptable to both chemical manufacturers and food processors. Furthermore, established specifications might well act as a guide in the development of new chemicals of a quality suitable for food use.

It is important that specifications for identity and quality of a food additive should be no more stringent than necessary to accomplish their purpose and that they should be reasonably attainable by the producing industries. Otherwise, the consuming public would ultimately bear an unnecessary additional cost of production and control (30-32).

Value in determining safety. One of the most important areas in which specifications for identity and purity would be of particular value is in the determination of the safety for use of food additives. It is essential to know the identity and concentration of the major component or components of a food additive before carrying out an effective toxicological investigation of its properties. Even small differences in composition of a compound may materially alter the results of toxicity tests. The investigator must also know the nature and quantity of the important impurities. Toxicologists have frequently emphasized that impurities or minor constituents may have a toxicological significance far greater than their amounts might indicate. Information relating to physical properties, such as solubility, is also essential.

In many animal tests, particularly with some of the relatively inert food additives, large amounts of the chemical are required and therefore the investigator must be certain that he has sufficient material of a uniform nature or a reliable source of the material of the same composition. In certain instances, years of animal studies have been discarded because the composition of the food additive changed during the test period. Furthermore, even if tests demonstrate beyond any reasonable doubt that a particular substance is safe for use, their value is impaired when the food additive used commercially differs significantly from the material tested.

The results of a single investigation are not likely to answer for all time the question of the safety for use of a particular material. Permitted additives should be subjected to continuing observation for possible deleterious effects under changing conditions of use and should be reappraised whenever indicated by advances in knowledge. Specifi-

cations based on the material used in previous tests would therefore
be of great value in making certain that a comparable product was
employed in such reappraisals. The divergent results which are occasionally encountered in the toxicological investigation of the same
product may conceivably be due to variations in the composition of
batches of the material under test (33,34).

In addition, specifications for food additives produced commercially
should be broad enough to include all the variations in the composition
of these additives that, according to current knowledge, do not significantly affect their biological properties. As an example, mono-
and di-glycerides of edible fatty acids are considered as coming under
one specification for the purpose of the toxicological evaluation. In
any case, each such group of additives will have to be judged individually with respect to the limits of composition set out in the specifications (35).

The problem of chemically related food additives has been examined
in several instances (36-39). The principle that each substance used as
a food additive should be considered separately has been followed as
far as identification is concerned In some cases, however, no differences in toxicology have been found between closely related substances--
for example, acids and their esters or salts--and one experimental
study may sometimes include work on several different compounds belonging to the same group. Although a separate specification should
be given for each substance, in appropriate cases related substances
might be considered jointly in the toxicological evaluation (40).

Since a number of food additives are closely related chemically and
toxicologically, a system of grouping food additives has been adopted.
The toxicological evaluation is expected to cover all the specified members of the group that may be included in the diet. In some cases, a
given food additive may be related to two groups, in which case the
level in the diet must not exceed the maximum acceptable level for
either group. The problem is not as complicated as it may appear at
first sight, since many of the substances in a group of additives are
likely to be used as alternatives to each other (39,41,42).

The relationship between chemical specifications and toxicological
aspects of a food additive is an important one because it brings into
the picture the problem of impurities, formulation, mixtures and composite products. It should be emphasized that adequate specifications
are extremely important in toxicological evaluations (43). This tends
to be the most neglected aspect and at times it may deceive scientists
by its apparent simplicity. In reality, adequate specifications are any-
thing but simple. A chemical name by itself is totally useless without
an accompanying definition of what is intended by that name. A food
additive is not a single compound but a commercial product that may
contain perhaps only 70% of the pure compound after which the product
is named; it may contain 90% or 95% but never 100%. For the purpose
of toxicological evaluations, the purity of a food additive may be ir-
relevant--the important considerations being only whether the purity
of the material used is consistent with the purity of the material that
was toxicologically tested. This aspect may present a number of dif-

ficulties. For example, materials that were tested many years ago may not have had adequate specifications and this may call into question the acceptability of the toxicological data because its relevance to the material manufactured at the present time is unknown. Furthermore, materials of different specifications may have been used for different parts of the testing program. These may be materials of different grades prepared by the same manufacturer or materials of similar grade but produced by different manufacturers using different processes. It follows that it is highly irresponsible to carry out new toxicological tests on food additives that are already in use without ensuring that the material used complies with the appropriate specifications (45).

In a number of instances the task of evaluating compounds that contain impurities or that give rise to transformation products of possible toxicological significance has presented itself.

The presence of harmful impurities in food additives can be excluded most effectively by the establishment of purity specifications. Food legislation should make provision for limits in foods of inorganic impurities such as arsenic and heavy metals. These requirements not only provide protection from the harmful effects of such contaminants, but also have a beneficial effect on the general level of food processing. On the other hand, some food additives may contain organic impurities which are particularly dangerous, the detection of which is difficult or impossible after admixture with food. In such instances it is most important that the specifications for the food additives should exclude or limit these substances (46).

The purity of a food additive refers to its freedom from substances other than those named in specifications. "Foreign substances" or "impurities" not included in the specifications may be, for example, simple inorganic salts or other substances not necessarily deleterious from the functional or safety standpoint.

Impurities may arise from the raw materials used in the manufacture of chemical (especially when they are complex natural substances), from substances used in processing steps, from solvents used in extraction or crystallization, or from equipment. They may also be unreacted intermediates or by-products formed in the course of processing, such as incompletely esterified acids or isomeric derivatives. Products of decomposition during storage, such as those which may result from oxidation, hydrolysis, or polymerization, are likewise regarded as impurities. However, the constituents of polymeric or other mixtures of reproducible composition are not regarded as impurities if they contribute to the functional properties of the substance as a whole and are not deleterious.

Obviously contaminants like dirt, soot, rust, lubricants and insect fragments must be avoided in manufacture, packaging, and storage of food additives. Whereas their presence is generally revealed in the application of the tests given in the specifications, no specific tests for the detection and identification of these contaminants are included.

From the foregoing discussion it is obvious that, depending on the original materials and manufacturing procedure, impurities may be volatile or nonvolatile, organic or inorganic, deleterious and nondeleterious. The important factors to be considered are:

a. Is the impurity one which might jeopardize the safe use of the food additive?
b. Is the amount of impurity sufficient to affect the activity or usefulness of the food additive?
c. Can the impurity be reduced in amount or avoided by good manufacturing practice?
d. Is the impurity of sufficient consequence to justify a limitation?

Whereas food additives are usually employed in relatively small quantities and traces of impurities may pose no serious health hazards, prudence dictates that reasonable limits be established for impurities consistent with good manufacturing practice as judged by modern standards (47).

Unique impurities and transformation products of possible toxicological significance may be classified into four categories on the basis of different modes of formation:

a. Unique impurities present by virtue of the manufacturing process e.g., 5-benzyl-3,6-dioxo-2-piperazine, (diketopiperazine, DKP) in aspartame, ortho-toluenesulfonamide in saccharin, cyclohexylamine in cyclamate, 4-methylimidazole in caramel produced by the ammonia process;

b. Transformation of the additive in food processing or storage, e.g., formation of DKP from aspartame, and fluorescein from erythrosine;

c. Reaction products with food constituents, e.g., formation of ethylurethane from diethyl pyrocarbonate, dichlorovinylcysteine from trichloroethylene, methionine sulfoximine from nitrogen trichloride, ethylene chlorhydrin from ethylene oxide, nitroso compounds from nitrites, tin compounds in certain canned products;

d. Metabolic transformation products, e.g., formation of cyclohexylamine from cyclamates, free aromatic amines from azo dyes, nitrites from nitrates.

It should be noted that certain food additives may contain impurities or give rise to transformation products as a result of more than one of the above mechanisms.

At an early stage in toxicological testing of food additives there is a need to consult with food technologists and chemists so as to be alerted to the possible occurrence of impurities or transformation products. Under certain circumstances an impurity or transformation product may have to be tested separately (48).

A food additive may be marketed as a formulated preparation consisting of a mixture of the main ingredient with a vehicle and possible other substances. Composite products such as enzyme preparations, contain one or more active components as well as diluents, preservatives, antioxidants and other substances used in food processing. While specifications are normally prepared for the pure substance that can be described in chemical terms, the variety of formulations used may not allow the drawing up of complete specifications for each individual product. In order to assure toxicological safety and the standard of purity required for such products in accordance with good manufacturing practice, general specifications may be prepared, setting out a number of criteria that would encompass all closely related products of the type in question. Whereever possible, additional requirements for individual products may be laid down in a specification. These are to be read in conjunction with the general specification.

Formulation does not affect the toxicological evaluation, provided that the substances added are known to be acceptable and that they do not alter the absorption or metabolism of the food additive in such a way that the biological data are thereby invalidated (49,50).

The question of microbiological contamination of food additives produced from natural sources and the need for the inclusion of some requirements in the specifications have been discussed on several occasions (51-54). Chemical specifications elaborated by the committee are spread over 14 volumes containing monographs of food additives considered during the 22 years of activity. No single document is available which would give a complete picture of the state of the art of this exercise. Since several of the relevant documents are no more available for distribution and since the character of documents involved makes it difficult at times to find the desired information, it has been recommended that the general principles governing the establishment of specifications should be reviewed in the light of the current work and future program of the committee and that suitable revised or edited specifications, together with the required methods of analysis, should be issued in a single compendium (55,56).

4. CONSIDERATIONS IN TOXICOLOGICAL TESTING PROCEDURES

4.1 General Scientific Background

During the last 23 years the Joint FAO/WHO Expert Committee on Food Additives has prepared 23 reports. Sixteen reports have resulted from the Joint FAO/WHO Meetings on Pesticide Residues and two general reports were elaborated by WHO Scientific Groups, all of which have been concerned with various aspects of the toxicology and safety evaluation of food additives, pesticides and chemicals in general that may be intentionally or unintentionally incorporated into food.

The significant advances of toxicology and of other fields relevant to these problems have led to discussions as to which testing procedures should be more suitable to provide evidence upon which decisions on safe use of food additives may be made.

Thus, for example, many new and more sensitive methods of analysis have been devised and applied to the detection of minute amounts of chemicals in the environment. The detailed study of metabolism at the molecular level has been applied to many problems and this has special relevance to toxicology. Modification of substances in the course of their metabolism may significantly affect their toxicity. Chemicals may alter enzyme activity and some substances may stimulate the production of metabolizing enzymes. Hence, for a full understanding of the effects of a chemical on biological systems, it is necessary to have as much knowledge as possible about the relationships between the chemical (and its derivatives) and the complex pattern of enzymes in living organisms.

Considerable advances have also been made in molecular biology, coupled with more detailed information on the structure and ultrastructure of cells and tissues--their relationship to function may now be interpreted in molecular terms. Various isolated fractions derived from cells and tissues can be subjected to detailed investigation. Electron microscopy and histochemistry are now commonly used in pathological and toxicological laboratories.

Important developments have occurred in the availability and quality of laboratory animals. Better genetic control, a wider range of species and the provision of animals in which common pathogens are controlled, or from which micro-organisms are completely eliminated, are also important to toxicologists.

These and other advances have resulted in the development of better methods of investigations in toxicology. It is now generally possible to study more precisely, or to follow in greater detail, the absorption, distribution, metabolism and elimination of a substance, to discover the modifications that may occur in the course of its passage through living systems, to investigate its effects on enzymes or morphology and to relate these observations to alterations in structure and function and to the signs and symptoms of toxicity. Thus, with increasing frequency, it should be possible to explain many toxicological phenomena in chemical and biochemical terms (57).

Scientists working in this field have a responsibility to indicate what whould be done to provide evidence for toxicological decisions. A well-designed study of the reactions of experimental animals to the administration of food additives, or the processed food itself, can provide the necessary evidence for making such decisions. However, the establishment of a uniform set of experimental procedures that would be standardized and obligatory is not only undesirable, since the satisfactory evolution of better methods depends upon the existence of full scientific freedom (58), it would also be unreasonable, as no single pattern of tests could adequately cover a range of substances so diverse in structure and function as food additives (59).

For the above-mentioned reasons, it is only possible to formulate general recommendations (58) or general guidelines (59) on testing procedures. Furthermore, it should be kept in mind that these guidelines are aimed at establishing the "safe use" of a chemical, not to study the toxicity per se or to study "toxicological procedures." Most scientists would agree that almost any chemical can be harmful at some dose and safe at another, although some workers maintain that there can be no safe level of dosage for proven carcinogens (60).

The procedures outlined below require all the resources of a well-equipped laboratory with an adequately trained staff having access to current scientific literature over a wide field. In particular it is essential that facilities exist for the housing of large numbers of small laboratory animals and for smaller numbers of other species. Competent staff in numbers sufficient for the proper care of the animals is also essential. The provision of such facilities on an adequate scale is very costly. These questions must be examined and adequate means made available before a laboratory is set up to undertake toxicological investigations. Preferably it should be situated in an environment where active research in allied fields is in progress (60).

The testing procedures indicated below are only a few among the many involved in toxicology and should be modified as necessary, depending on the nature of the substance to be tested, and should take advantage of recent developments in toxicological techniques (61).

4.2 Experimental Animals

4.2.1 Generalities

The successful use of experimental animals depends upon the care taken in their selection and maintenance throughout the experiment. It is important to have a well-designed animal house with adequate ventilation and temperature control.

As much as possible should be known about the normal duration of life and the incidence of natural disease, tumors in particular, in the animals used in long-term studies. Such information is necessary in order that the significance of any disease in the experimental groups can be assessed. For this reason rats or mice from a known strain, either bred in the laboratory or obtained from the same commercial breeder, should be used so that such information can be gradually assembled. In other species, the age and previous history of the animals should be known where possible.

For feeding tests, rats should preferably be housed singly, and given a basic diet of consistent composition adequate to support growth and reproduction under ordinary conditions. When the investigator wishes to examine toxicity under conditions of dietary deficiency, a special diet will obviously be needed. The routine use of inadequate diets in investigations of the toxicity of a food additive is, however, not recommended.

Before starting a toxicological investigation, careful consideration should be given to the experimental design to ensure that, by means of the proper statistical treatment, the maximum amount of information may be extracted from the data. Whenever measurements are made of differences between the control and experimental animals, the significance of such differences should be estimated statistically (62).

4.2.2 Appropriate Species

It is often stated that results obtained in the most sensitive species should take precedence in toxicological evaluation. However, it is recommended that, whenever possible, the most appropriate species should be chosen for this purpose. This would be the species most similar to man with regard to its metabolic, biochemical and toxicological characteristics in relation to the substance under test (63).

In carcinogenicity testing particularly, both sexes of each of at least two species of animals should be used in the tests throughout their life span. In most cases these species would be rats and mice. Hamsters or dogs might be suitable, but guinea-pigs, for example, appear to be resistant to some known carcinogens. The use of dogs in carcinogenicity tests has disadvantages. Because of the expense of their maintenance, it is difficult to use a sufficient number to detect a low incidence of cancer, and the life span of a dog is 12-15 years.

The animals used should be bred in the laboratory in which the tests are carried out. The characteristics of the colony, including sensitivity to carcinogens, should be known, and the incidence of spontaneous tumors should be recorded. Out-bred or random-bred animals are generally acceptable. If pure strains are used then at least two strains should be employed. There are advantages in using F_1 hybrids of two pure strains of animals.

The treatment should begin when the animals are young--in the case of rodents, soon after weaning. Animals should be kept under good conditions and should be as free as possible from parasites or infectious diseases, especially those that may shorten the life span or may lead to tumor production (64).

4.2.3 Number of Experimental Animals

A major difficulty arises in connection with the number of animals needed in order to obtain reasonable confidence limits within which the failure to detect an effect may be expressed. The application of relevant statistical principles indicates the need to use several hundred animals at each dose level in order to assure with reasonable probability that the occasional reactor--e. g. 1 in 100--may be observed in any experiment. Even so it may be very difficult to detect such an abnormal reactor and impossible to attribute the effect to the material under test. It is unrealistic to suggest the use of such large numbers. Instead, reliance can be placed on an ability to observe a response in the majority of the animals receiving dose levels far in excess of those recommended for human consumption (65).

Particularly in carcinogenicity testing the number of animals in each group should be sufficient to yield statistically reliable results. For example, where no tumors appear in the control group there must be at least four tumors in the experimental group for the result to be considered significant at a P value of 0.025 (see the tabulation on facing page):

In most cases, however, tumors develop also in the control group. Table I gives the relative incidences necessary for a difference between the two groups to be significant for a P value of 0.05. This can be applied to each type of tumor separately or to the sum of all tumors observed in each group, if the tumor types are similar and therefore comparable. The establishment of negative results, particularly im-

Number of animals in each group	Minimum percentage incidence in experimental groups that can be regarded as significant (P=0.025)*
4	100.0
6	66.7
10	40.0
15	26.7
20	20.0
25	16.0
30	13.3
35	11.4
50	8.0
75	5.3
100	4.0

*Where no tumors appear in controls, and where equal numbers of control and experimental animals reach tumor-bearing age (66).

portant in the investigation of food additives, presents more difficulty. Even with reasonable confidence limits it would be necessary to use several hundreds of animals per experimental group to exclude the chance occurrence of a 1% incidence of tumors above the incidence in the control group. As noted above, it is unrealistic to suggest the use of such large numbers. Instead, it is necessary to rely on the fact that a response in a higher percentage of the animals is to be expected if dose levels are used far in excess of those recommended for human consumption.

Since a long induction period often precedes the appearance of tumors, consideration should be given to expected mortality so that a sufficient number of survivors remains for evaluation. In the case of negative response, at least 20 animals of each sex should survive for two years with rats and 80 weeks with mice in each of the different groups (67).

4.2.4 Diet

The basal diet used in any toxicological feeding study should be palatable and nutritionally complete for the species under investigation, permitting normal growth, reproduction and life span. However, excessive amounts of any essential nutrient should be avoided. Full details of the composition of the basal diet should always be reported and in order to allow direct control over its uniformity, the diet should preferably be prepared in the investigator's own laboratory. When commercial rations are used, their composition with respect to both the ingredients and the nutrient levels should be known and satisfactory assurance should be obtained of their constancy of composition. In investigations for carcinogenicity, it is essential to avoid contamination of diets and cages with insecticides, disinfectants, or detergents, and in the case of commercial pelleted diets, traces of lubricants.

TABLE I (68)

Differences between two groups necessary for significance at a P value of 0.05*

50 animals per group		40 animals per group		30 animals per group		20 animals per group		10 animals per group	
Number less affected**	Number more affected	Number less affected	Number more affected	Number less affected	Number more affected	Number less affected	Number more affected	Number less affected	Number more affected
0	6	0	6	0	6	0	6	0	5
2	8	2	8	1	8	1	7	1	7
5	13	4	11	3	11	2	9	2	8
10	19	8	17	6	14	4	11	3	9
15	25	12	21	9	17	6	13	4	10
20	30	16	25	12	20	8	15	5	10
25	35	20	29	15	23	10	17	6	--
30	40	24	33	18	26	12	18	7	--
35	44	28	36	21	28	14	20	8	--
40	47	32	38	24	30	16	--	9	--
45	--	36	--	27	--	18	--		

*This table applies only to each type of tumor separately.
**"Less affected" generally refers to control group.

To permit accurate recording of food consumption, diets should be in dry form, but if this is not possible owing to the moist or fluid nature of the test material, special precautions must be taken to ensure adequate measurement of intake. The effect of oxidative rancidity of fat components should be reduced by incorporating them at weekly or more frequent intervals, by storing under refrigeration fats, oils and diets containing them, and by frequent replenishment of the feed cups.

Test materials should not be incorporated in diets if they are unstable or likely to react with any of their components. In such cases direct oral or intragastric administration may be employed provided the control animals are treated similarly with a placebo. When test substances are mixed into the ration, uniform distribution should be assured. If a solvent or vehicle is necessary, it should be incorporated into the control diet. No solvent that leaves residue upon evaporation should be used:

When test materials are incorporated into the ration of young, rapidly growing rats, cognizance must be taken of the diminution in food intake relative to body-weight. This also applies to female rats during pregnancy. In order to maintain uniformity of dosage during this period the concentration of test material in the diet may be adjusted as indicated in Table II.

TABLE II

Example of dietary adjustment to maintain uniform dosage level

Dose	Period after weaning at 3 weeks (weeks)	Food intake (g/kg day)	(% of the diet)
100 mg/kg of body-weight	0.2	120	0.084
	2-4	100	0.100
	4-6	75	0.133
	6-8	65	0.154
	8-10	60	0.168
	10+	50	0.200

Throughout a lifetime study, periodic records of food consumption, taken at appropriate intervals with representative animals from each test and control group, should provide the basis for checking the actual dosages of test substances consumed (69).

4.2.5 Tests by the Oral Route

4.2.5.1 Selection of Dosage Range

Doses should be selected carefully so that the maximum amount of
information may be obtained. Tumor formation may be restricted to
dosage levels which produce other chronic toxic effects or may be
demonstrable at one or more lower levels. It is advisable, therefore,
to select as many and as wide a range of doses as may be possible.

As a guide to selection of the dosage level of the agent under study,
the investigator should consult available information upon its short-
term (sub-acute) toxicity. If little is known about the toxicity of the
test material it is preferable to do a range-finding experiment before
doses are selected (70). The highest dose used for determination of
carcinogenicity should be one which produced a minimal to moderate
amount of short-term toxicity. This may be described as the maximum
dose for measurement of carcinogenic activity. If only one other dose
is to be used, a level of 1/4 to 1/3 the maximum dose may be employed. If three doses are chosen, multiples of 1, 1/3 and 1/9 the
maximum dose are suggested. It is important to aim at including a
dose that does not materially decrease the life span.

From the data on acute oral toxicity, information upon short-term
toxicity may be approximated (68). It may also be possible to obtain
satisfactory doses for measurement of carcinogenicity from the data
on acute oral toxicity alone. One method is to begin with daily doses
of 5%, 10% and 20% of the oral LD_{50}. If one or more of these doses
produces short-term toxicity reactions, then all three daily doses are
halved or otherwise lowered. If no short-term toxicity reactions appear,
then all doses are doubled or otherwose increased By this method an
approximate dose-response curve may be obtained (71).

4.2.5.2 Methods of Administration

Daily oral doses may be given in food, drinking-water, or by intragastric intubation. Test materials are usually incorporated in the diet,
and the concentration is adjusted so that the expected daily intake contains the dose required. The percentage to be added to food may be
recalculated as indicated by changes in the daily consumption of food,
which may be estimated at weekly or other intervals as suggested in
Table II. The dosage may be expressed as a concentration in the diet,
in which case the food intake of the groups must be relatively uniform
or known. An excess of this food mixture is given to permit the animals to eat ad libitum.

The daily dose may be given dissolved in drinking-water by a similar method of calculation. The solution should be changed daily and the
water bottles kept thoroughly clean.

Giving the daily dose by gastric intubation permits more exact measurement of dosage. The dose should be dissolved, suspended, or
emulsified and given in relation to body-weight.

4.2.5.3 Control Groups

The incidence, time of appearance, number and type of tumor which may be found in the treated groups must be compared statistically with corresponding data in control animals. The control groups must be treated in a manner identical to that used in the dosage groups except that they are not exposed to the agent under study, neither must they be exposed to carcinogenic contaminants. The control group should be at least as large as the test group. If many test groups are involved, the size of the control group may be calculated as $\overline{N}$ x number of animals per dosage group, when N equals the number of dosage groups (e. g. , 100 controls for four dosage groups of 50 animals per dosage group). In special cases, positive control groups may be used which are given appropriate carcinogens for the purpose of comparison (72).

4.2.6 Tests by Parenteral Routes

4.2.6.1 Skin Applications

Test materials are applied in solvents which should be non-irritant and free from carcinogenic contaminants. Acetone is considered suitable for many materials. The concentration of the test material should be as high as possible so that a small volume is applied. The back of the mouse and the ear of the rabbit are sites commonly used for this type of test. The material may be applied one to three times per week for a period of at least a year and the animals should be observed for their lifetime.

4.2.6.2 Subcutaneous Injection

Only solvents which are non-irritant and not contaminated with carcinogens should be used, and control groups of animals must be injected with the solvent only. If an adqueous solution is injected, the osmotic pressure and the pH should approximate to physiological values. For lipid-soluble materials, non-fluorescent tricaprylin or molecularly distilled triolein may be used. Injections should be given at weekly or monthly intervals for up to one year. The volume of each injection should be small to reduce the incidence of irrelevant effects. Insoluble materials can be injected as suspensions in suitable vehicles.

4.2.6.3 Intraperitoneal and Intramuscular Injection

Injection into the peritoneal cavity or into muscle might have advantages as compared with injection into subcutaneous tissue. These methods, however, need further investigation before they can be evaluated (73).

4.2.7 Examination of the Animals

Regular and frequent determinations of body weight and food intake give a measure of the condition of the animals. It is of great value to have experienced personnel make frequent and regular clinical examinations of the animals. In this way cannibalism, for example, can be avoided. Moribund animals should be killed.

A complete post-mortem examination should be performed. The entire alimentary tract should be opened and organs often ignored (e.g., the pituitary) should be inspected whenever possible. Scientists trained in pathology and familiar with the diseases of laboratory animals, particularly tumors, should perform the autopsies or at least supervise these examinations. All organs showing macroscopic lesions should be examined histopathologically (74).

4.2.7.1 Well-defined Effects

Data on death of the animals, convulsions or other well-defined effects can usually be expressed quantitatively and it may be possible to calculate the effective dose for 50% of the animals treated (ED_{50}). The statistical significance of such observations should be assessed.

4.2.7.2 Differences in Weight Gain

If a statistically significant difference in weight gain is found, it is essential that food intake should be checked. If the differences in weight gain can be fully accounted for by the differences in food intake, the result may be attributable either to anorexia or lack of palatability of the experimental diet need not be relevant to the health hazard involved.

4.2.7.3 Nutritional Effects

If food intake differences do not account for differences in weight gain, appropriate studies should be carried out to determine whether absorption or utilization of food materials is at fault, or some impairment of their nutritional value has taken place. The nature and extent of any significant nutritional damage should be separately defined by appropriate assay procedures.

4.2.7.4 Study of Different Organs

Functional tests: Functional tests are available for the study of the gastro-intestinal, hepatic, renal, haematopoietic, nervous and reproductive systems and can be applied to some of the common laboratory animals. Tests may be of two types, i.e., relatively simple screening tests, or more complex studies in which the different aspects of the function may be separately analyzed. They provide useful quantitative information, but it must be remembered that vital organs commonly possess a considerable reserve so that functional inadequacy may not be apparent until appreciable damage has occurred.

Macroscopic appearance: Careful and critical autopsy is important. The observations made cannot be readily measured quantitatively, but they serve as indices of the need for more detailed study.

Relative organ weights: Organ weights, related to body weight or some other common index, can be compared in experimental and control groups. Statistically significant differences indicate the need for more detailed study. Such differences, however, do not necessarily indicate, nor does their absence exclude, the existence of any deleterious effect.

Histopathology: Differences in microscopical appearances may be the earliest detectable sign of toxicity. Instances have been reported in which the histopathological method was the only one that revealed a deleterious effect. The importance of histopathological studies in this field is, therefore, apparent. On the other hand, it is only an extremely small proportion of the vast numbers of microscopical preparations that has provided useful positive data in the toxicological studies on food additives. Every effort should be made to reduce the load of routine histopathological examination in these studies by improving the simpler and less time-consuming observations, such as macroscopic appearance and organ weights, so that critical histopathological study may eventually be restricted to those occasions on which it will be of the greatest value.

4.2.7.5 Organs Likely to Yield Useful Data

Organs of elimination: The main organs of elimination, the kidneys, liver and gastro-intestinal tract should be subjected to appropriate study.

Hematopoietic and reproductive systems: While these tissues have an importance in their own right, they are perhaps of special interest in the investigations under discussion because they are the sites of active cell proliferation and their study may consequently assist in the elucidation of cytotoxic effects.

Other organs: Where there is any special indication of possible effects in other organs, such as the thyroid or the brain, appropriate investigations should be carried out (75).

4.2.8 Duration of Toxicity Tests

For adequate interchange of information, a precise description is more meaningful than such terms as "acute," "subacute," "short-term" and "chronic." Each report of an experiment should state in precise terms, in respect of both control and test animals, the species, sex, diet, route of administration and duration. The objective should be to define clearly all the known variables.

Scientific judgement is necessary in determining the duration of animal studies for the evaluation of an individual food additive. Where adequate biochemical and toxicological data on closely related chemicals are available, the objective becomes the detection of any deviation from the established pattern. This can usually be determined by intensive studies of a few months' duration when these are adequately designed and evaluated. Appropriate studies in humans add significantly to the adequacy of the data.

In the absence of such definitive data, or if there are reasons to suspect carcinogenic potential, longer-germ studies must still be relied upon for reassurance. Recent advances in the quality of research animals, and particularly in the control of pathogens, have increased the life-span of some strains of animals. In spite of this, feeding studies adequately designed and evaluated extending up to eighteen months in mice and two years in rats are still considered adequate to ensure a minimum safeguard in evaluating the carcinogenic potential of a chemical additive. In special cases it may be desirable to prolong the observations in these species.

If there are good reasons to doubt the relevance to man of the data obtained in rodent species--for example, if the metabolism of the additive in man is found to be significantly different from that in rodents-- it may be desirable to carry out investigations of longer duration in other species. The design and conduct of reproduction and teratogenic studies should take into account placental and mammary transmission. In addition, the investigation of some potential toxic effects, particularly carcinogenicity, requires careful prolonged observation of the offspring. Detailed study of general appearance and behavior, biochemical effects, metabolism and histopathology should be included and fully reported, both qualitatively and quantitatively (76).

In conclusion, flexibility of approach is essential in deciding the duration of tests necessary to establish that a compound is safe. In certain circumstances, tests carried out over a few months may suffice for the purpose of detecting any deviation from the established pattern in a group of closely related chemicals (77).

The fact that additives may be taken over the greater part of a lifetime gives rise to concern lest such prolonged intake may produce reactions hitherto unsuspected. The possibilities that any such reaction may follow the ingestion of food additives can best be examined experimentally by feeding much higher doses of the material to animals during the greater part, or the whole, of their lifetimes. In the absence of any indication to the contrary, such prolonged tests must form a part of any experimental work designed to supply evidence in support of a claim for the safe use of a food additive (78).

New approaches and new techniques make it now possible to probe in depth into the nature of the earliest response of the organism to exposure to a chemical. The interpretation of observations is often difficult and is not made easier by the administration of high doses in studies on substances of relatively low toxic potential. There are also instances where adaptive changes occur. Since many toxicological decisions are based on the assessment of the highest dose level that causes no deleterious effect, the differentiation of adverse effects from other changes is crucial (79).

4.2.9 Toxicity and Nutritional Status

Nutritional status can influence toxicity. The effects of starvation or more specific nutritional dificiencies on the biological response to different substances will vary widely. It has been shown, for example, that glycogen depletion in the liver may interfere with the production of metabolizing enzymes in mice and in guinea-pigs (80,81). Poor nutritional status does not necessarily increase susceptibility to toxic effects. For example, depression of metabolizing enzymes that give rise to toxic products may diminish susceptibility. The general effects of reduced food intake on biological responses have been reviewed by Friedman (82), and the effects of specific nutritional deficiencies on toxicity have been fully discussed by Hotzel (83).

The composition of the intestinal flora and such practices as coprophagy have an important influence on the nutritional status of experimental animals.

Carcinogenic action tends to be diminished by caloric restriction and protein deficiency and in certain cases by specific nutritional deficiencies.

The relationship between nutritional status and carcinogenesis has been reviewed by Tannenbaum (84) and discussed in WHO reports (86).

So far as toxicity studies are concerned, it is wise to maintain all the animals on a diet that is nutritionally adequate in every way, unless there is some specific reason for doing otherwise. It follows from the complexity of the effects of starvation or specific nutritional deficiencies in different species of animals that the indiscriminate use of undernutrition or dietary deficiences might give rise to misleading results. A clear distinction must be drawn between investigations forming part of research projects and toxicological studies intended for safety evaluation. In applying the results of such safety tests, the state of nutrition of the individuals exposed is taken into account by means of appropriate adjustments in the margin of safety used in specific instances. Equally, such adjustments must make allowance for other relevant factors in the chemical environment to which the population under consideration is exposed.

Food additives may be used, or contamination of food with chemicals may occur, in countries in which malnutrition is widespread. Further work is needed on the effects of various states of malnutrition or undernutrition on the toxicity manifested by chemical compounds.

Manipulation of the composition of the diet of experimental animals, either in an effort to simulate conditions of malnutrition in man or in the belief that such dietary modifications help to elicit latent toxic effects of the material under study, is not considered advisable in routine toxicological investigations intended for the evaluation of safety (87).

In conclusion, because of the complexity of the relationships between nutritional state and toxicity, at present the evaluation of safety is best carried out by using healthy animals on adequate balanced diets (88).

4.2.10 Effect of Age on Toxicity

The response of an animal to a particular substance may vary with age. In general, but not invariably, the young animal is more sensitive to the toxic effects of exposure to chemicals. The difference may arise from the presence of distinctive flora in the upper part of the bowel, a factor that accounts for the susceptibility of human babies to poisoning by nitrates. In most cases, however, there exists an enzymic basis for the age difference in response to foreign compounds.

Many foreign substances are metabolized in the body by enzymes that occur in the endoplasmic reticulum of the liver cells. There is evidence that these enzymes may be poorly developed in newborn animals possibly owing to lack of inducers. Here also there may be significant species differences. In the rat the activity of the group of enzymes commonly called "drug-metabolizing enzymes" and mainly studies in the liver is maximal at the age of about 30 days and thereafter declines to some extent. Glucuronyl transferase is deficient in many newborn animals, including man, but not in the rat.

Thus, the enzymes that metabolize foreign substances may be at a low level in newborn animals but develop later. Occasionally, they may be found in the newborn of some species, but not of others. A few metabolizing enzymes may be present in the newborn of some species although enzyme activity is no longer manifest in the adult animal of the same species. In any case, the metabolizing enzymes may either enhance or diminish toxicity, depending upon the biological properties of the substrate and the various products, although in the main these enzymes act beneficially.

These considerations must be applied to the question of the possible presence of additives or trace contaminants in the diets of babies. It should be stressed that, in spite of the often considerable efforts made by manufacturers to avoid the presence of contaminants in baby foods, under present-day conditions the diet of babies is likely to contain traces of pesticide and other residues. In addition, there are circumstances in which the benefit to the baby arising from the inclusion of some additive, for example a preservative, in its diet may greatly outweigh any possible hazard. Nevertheless, it is necessary to exercise great care in making such additions, keeping in mind the possible long duration of exposure.

Since babies constitute a special population, close observation of epidemiology in this group is an important practical aspect of the evaluation of effects of exposure. The need exists for further information on the development of enzyme systems in the human young, with particular emphasis on those enzymes responsible for dealing with foreign compounds (89).

Very young infants are especially vulnerable to foreign chemicals because the mechanisms that provide protection against these substances are absent or not fully developed. Although the evidence for this derives mainly from studies with drugs rather than with food additives, it is likely that such very young infants are less efficient than older children in metabolizing some food additives and may therefore accumulate them to excessive levels. If this occurs at a time when sensitivity to toxic effects is critical because of the delicately balanced growth and differentiation processes, there may be deleterious consequences that may not appear until much later in the child's development. Very young infants may also differ from older children in relation to physiological barriers protecting sensitive tissues, such as the blood-brain barrier or the protective barriers for retinal or lens tissue.

The known differences between the very young infant and the older child include the following: low gastric acid secretion, different biochemical capabilities of the gastrointestinal tract, inability to digest and absorb certain substances, deficiency in methaemaglobin reductase systems, and diminished renal excretory processes at both glomerular and tubular sites (90).

Modifications into some of the recommended procedures for all toxicological testing of intentional and unintentional food additives should be introduced when the additive is designed to be included in infant foods.

Before a food additive is regarded as safe for use in food intended for infants up to 12 weeks of age, the toxicological studies should be extended to include animals in the corresponding period of life. There is, however, a lack of precise information relating to this developmental period in both animals and the human infant. It is difficult to recommend precise toxicological testing procedures until more basic research has been undertaken. There are also difficulties in selecting the appropriate species. In these circumstances short-term studies should be conducted in several species and should include the oral administration of the additive under test, at suitable dose levels, to newly born animals up to and including the end of the weaning period. This type of exposure is necessary in order to discover whether the existing species variation seriously affects the handling of the food additive by the test animals and to compensate partly for the serious lack of knowledge in this area both in animals and men.

When life span studies and multigeneration studies are carried out, they should be extended to include the oral administration of the food additive at suitable dose levels to a proportion of animals from the day of birth throughout the pre-weaning period. These animals should then be observed for the required period as laid down for the usual life span and multigeneration tests should be carried out for at least three generations. If there are any indications of heritable mutagenic effects, these tests should be followed by specific studies. Some members of the filial generations should be exposed to the additive for their lifespan. The enchanced sensitivity of the newborn of several species to certain carcinogenic agents is particularly relevant in this regard. It is also necessary to place greater emphasis in future on observations of the behavioral developments of animals used for toxicological testing, particularly in long-term studies. Because of uncertainties still existing in this field, the accumulation of experimental information is of paramount importance for the evaluation of the results in terms of human health hazard (91).

4.2.11 Exposure in utero and Post-natal Period

More recently, in discussing the physiological factors that may explain the higher sensitivity of newborn and young infants, it was observed that the same factors are of even greater importance for the embryo in utero. Hitherto, toxicological studies have been mainly concerned with embryotoxic effects that manifest themselves by fetal lethality and with teratogenic effects recognizable at birth and during the immediate post-natal period. It has become evident in recent years that exposure to toxic chemicals in utero may have effects that cannot be recognized during these developmental stages but appear later in life as tumors, changes in immunological mechanisms, and disturbances of behavior and neurological functions.

In order to gain more information about the long-term effects of exposure to chemicals in utero and in the post-natal period, appropriate toxicological methodology must be developed. The problem of transplacental carcinogenesis as a potential long-term effect has been already discussed in the past (1). While it has been observed that this is an important problem, attention was also drawn to other possible long-term effects such as changes in behavior and immunological mechanism. Since the experimental approach to these problems may depend on the chemical, toxicological and pharmacokinetic properties of the compound, no specific toxicological protocol was proposed. However, it was emphasized that the short- and long-term effects of exposure in utero and during the lactation period should be taken into account when evaluating food additives and contaminants. This evaluation might include a request for appropriate animal studies (234).

The question of feeding studies employing the progeny of exposed parents was further discussed subsequently and it was noted that several expert groups have discussed the desirability of recommending long-term feeding studies in which animals are exposed to the agent under study in utero and during suckling (234, 237).

It was agreed that such studies would assist in evaluating the potential hazards of food additives or contaminants consumed by child-bearing women. These studies would also broaden the scope of toxicological assessment generally (238). However, there have been only limited applications of this approach so far. Furthermore, the approach presents significant technical and logistic difficulties. Because of the complexity of this important and rapidly developing field and because of its significance to the public health, it was recommended that WHO should explore the means of convening a meeting of experts to draw up guidelines for studies. The experts should be requested specifically to:

a. Assess:
   1. the degree of the possible increase in sensitivity of toxicological testing afforded by exposure in utero and through lactation;
   2. the need to include such exposure in toxicological tests as a means of increasing public health protection;

b. Propose the most appropriate guidelines for experimentation taking into account:
   1. The dosage levels used and the relative exposures of mother and foetus to the agent under study;
   2. the posibility of combining this modified long-term test with reproduction studies;
   3. the length of the studies required; and
   4. the most appropriate species which should be employed.

In the meantime, in the case of certain substances, it was agreed that requirements for such studies would be based on the best judgment and made in the light of existing data and other information that indicated their desirability (236).

Further problems may arise when aged animals are used for the evaluation of safety. It is better to carry out toxicity studies before the complications of senescence arise. It is clearly essential in all such investigations to record the age of the animals as one of the factors of major importance in the experimental design (92).

In summary, as far as animal experimentation is concerned, it may be stated that by and large the young animal is more sensitive to the toxic effects of exposure to chemicals, but this is not invariably so. Useful information may be obtained from studies in newborn or young animals, from reproduction studies and from biochemical studies (88).

4.3 Substance to be Tested

Before toxicity tests are undertaken, the investigator must be certain that the material supplied for testing has the same specifications as that which will subsequently be used commercially. He must also know the nature and quantity of the more important impurities, since these may represent a greater health hazard than the additive itself. The chemical nature and physical properties of the substance under test may guide the investigator in the design of his experiments since they may indicate possible pathways of absorption and metabolism, as well as likely biological effects.

It should be emphasized, however, that the toxic or other biological effects of the test material cannot be predicted solely from a consideration of its chemical and physical properties.

Food additives are usually substances that cause some change in the properties of food materials. While the changes that are intentionally induced in this way should be to the advantage of the consumer, it is clearly necessary to ensure that other concomitant changes are not disadvantageous. The nature of the probably reactions with food materials can often be predicted and appropriate investigations should be planned to define any significant changes that may occur. These changes may be of two types. The first is concerned with modification of nutritional value. This should be studied by direct measurement of the appropriate nutrients by suitable chemical or biological assay methods. The second is the formation of new and possibly toxic substances by the modification of food ingredients. Changes in the test substance consequent upon cooking, storage or the application of other procedures, including changes which may result from its addition to the diets of the experimental animals, must also be borne in mind. These points must be studied if necessary, by the toxicological investigation of treated food materials. A safety factor may be introduced in this type of experiment by giving the animals food deliberately overtreated to a measured extent.

If the amount of the substance added to food has to fall within specified limits, an adequate method of quantitative assessment is essential. If details of a method of isolation and analysis of the test material that is effective when applied to the finished product can be provided at the outset, investigation and acceptance may be greatly facilitated. It is sometimes overlooked that no accurate assessment of the hazard attending the use of a substance, even though it is of known toxicity, can be made unless the quantities present in food can be measured (93).

It is therefore essential that adequate specifications for identity and purity should be available before toxicological work is initiated. Toxicologists and regulatory bodies need assurance that the material to be tested corresponds to that to be used in practice. Ideally, the specifications should be such as to define a material that will give reproducible biological results.

Specifications for food additives produced commercially should be broad enough to include all the variations in the composition of these additives that, according to current knowledge, do not significantly affect their biological properties.

Specifications for food additives produced commercially should be broad enough to include all the variations in the composition of these additives that, according to current knowledge, do not significantly affect their biological properties.

The levels of impurities that, according to current knowledge, are considered to be toxicologically significant and the methods for their determination must appear in the specifications. Tests for impurities such as lead, arsenic and heavy metals as a measure of good manufacturing practice should be maintained, unless and until a better measure becomes available. These tests are needed, irrespective of the high standards usually maintained in manufacture, in cases where inexperienced and less well-equipped manufacturers may produce food additives (94).

The remarks on chemical and physical specifications reported above also apply to special studies for carcinogenic activity of food additives. Important aspects are that samples to be tested should be representative of the composition of the material intended for human use, and that the chemical and physical properties used in identification of the samples (e.g. absorption spectra or chromatographic analyses) be reported in detail.

It is desirable to obtain and preserve one sample for the complete test, but if the material is unstable, or if, for other reasons, it is necessary to use samples from different batches, then each fresh supply should be carefully checked for identity. Sufficient information on vapor pressure and stability should be available to decide whether or not the material can be administered to the animals by mixing it into the diet or into the drinking water, and how frequently such mixtures should be prepared.

The identity of samples to be used for the testing of food contaminants presents difficulties, particularly when the exact composition of the contaminant is not known. For instance, some pesticide residues may be present mainly as break-down or reaction products. In preparing samples for testing, such possible changes should be taken into account. In special cases it may be necessary to test the treated food product as a whole instead of the original pesticide or its known reaction products (95).

4.4 Metabolic and Biochemical Investigations

Several types of study are included under this heading. Significant biochemical aspects include mode, rate and degree of absorption, levels of storage in organs and tissues, metabolic transformation, and mode and rate of elimination. Modifications of substances during metabolism may significantly affect their toxicity. Knowledge of whether or not a food additive is rapidly metabolized into innocuous degradation products or is rapidly excreted or accumulated in certain organs or tissues may be of great value in assessing potential hazards (96,97).

It is important to know whether a substance is absorbed, what factors may affect its absorption, how the substance is distributed in the body, where and how it is metabolized, and the route by which it is eliminated. Such information is by no means always available.

In evaluating the toxicological status of a substance it may be helpful to know the metabolic pathways that it follows in the body, and whether the changes in structure that take place during metabolism result in any significant change in the biological effects of the substance (98).

The aspect of metabolic and biochemical activity that might be profitably studied include the route and rate of absorption of the test material, the levels of storage in the tissues, and the subsequent fate of the stored material. Studies of the metabolism of the material, together with the identification of the metabolites, might be extended to include balance experiments in which an attempt is made to account for the administrered dose as metabolites excreted or material stored in the body. These studies would be done in the first instance with high dosage levels and should be extended to include doses nearer the levels proposed in food and the study of the effects of continuous administration. Other investigations might include the examination of enzymic processes which may be affected, the effect of additives on the nutritive value of the diet, and the possibility of the formation of toxic substances during processing, storage and household preparation.

In some cases it may be desirable, in order to learn more about the mode of action, to carry out certain studies in which pharmacodynamic techniques are used. Such investigations might well reveal effects which are not apparent in the short- and long-term feeding tests-- for instance, effects on the cardiovascular, autonomic, nervous or reproductive systems (99).

In biochemical studies, the possibility of reactions of the additive with food constituents should be taken into account. As noted earlier, such reactions are of two types. First, the nutritional value of the food may be affected. This possibility may be studied by chemical or biological assay methods. Second, new and possibly toxic substances may be formed. These must be investigated by the usual toxicological procedures. Cooking, storage, or the application of other technicological procedures may also alter the test substance. It may be necessary to undertake a toxicological investigation of treated food materials. Here a margin of safety may be introduced by conducting the tests with food that has been deliberately overtreated to a measured extent (100).

There are examples of a major metabolite being inactive and a minor one being more active than the original material from which both were derived. Balance studies in which all the metabolites have to be accounted for are much more difficult than the usual study in which the identification of one or two metabolites is all that is accomplished. It may be desirable to carry out such balance studies on food additives but this would be a formidable undertaking.

Most metabolic studies must be done at high dosage levels in the first instance, if the experimenter is to have any chance of isolating the metabolites. Metabolic processes are influenced by the size of the dose, and the proportion of the dose excreted as a particular metabolite may vary at different dosage levels (101).

Biochemical studies on food additives are long-term projects involving basic research and they are unlikely to replace the chronic toxicity test in the foreseeable future (101). However, an adequate knowledge of the metabolism and biochemical effects of a food additive has provided in some cases a satisfactory basis for recommending its use or rejection (99). Furthermore, some additives may be converted into substances already present naturally in food in much greater amounts. If the biochemical evidence shows that the sole effect of the additive is to make a small contribution to existing metabolic loads from food components, there is no need for detailed toxicological studies (100).

In addition, it may be possible to dispense with elaborate long-term studies if it can be convincingly shown that the substance is not absorbed or is broken down completely before absorption into well-known substances that are generally recognized as having no deleterious action. In any case, a proper understanding of the changes that the food additive may undergo in the food, in the gastro-intestinal tract, or in the body is necessary for the full interpretation of the biological and toxicological data (102).

If a series of chemical analogues can be shown to give rise to the same main metabolic product and to other compounds that are already present in the organism in greater quantities, or that can be readily and safely metabolized, it may be sufficient to carry out toxicological studies on a suitable representative of the series (100).

Any food additive that is completely broken down in the food or in the gastro-intestinal tract to substances that are common dietary or body constituents might be satisfactorily evaluated with respect to safety-in-use on the basis of appropriate biochemical and metabolic studies alone, without the necessity for the usual toxicological investigations. It was considered that the carrying out of extensive toxicological investigation of small amounts of common food constituents with the object of establishing the safety of their use as food additives was an unwarranted waste of scientific effort (103).

Finally, it is highly important that information about the metabolism and distribution of a substance undergoing testing should be obtained at an early stage since it may then be possible to make similar investigations in man. The information from such investigations will make it possible to choose, for further experimentation. The animal species corresponding most closely to man in the absorption and metabolism

of the substance and thus to obtain data on animal toxicity that will enhance predictive value (100).

4.5 Enzyme Studies

The effects of the additive on important enzyme systems in blood
or tissues should be studied. For example, an increase in the level
of certain marker enzymes in the serum, such as transaminases and
other intracellular enzymes, may be indicative of tissue damage. Another aspect to be investigated is the induction of microsomal enzyme
systems, especially in the liver. The relevance to man of these biochemical changes needs careful assessment (104).

The study of enzymes in relation to pharmacological and toxicological action has developed considerably in recent years. Increases
or decreases in enzyme levels caused by foreign chemicals may be
studied either in the blood or in the tissues. It has become more and
more apparent that, among the action mechanisms of toxic substances,
those of a biochemical nature are of prime importance. In this connection, the basic enzyme systems are certainly among the first sites
of action to merit careful study, since their inhibition often constitutes
the casual biochemical lesion that determines, at least in part, the
nature of toxic effects. Among other classical examples, it is enough
to recall the inhibiting effect of cyanides and sulfides on cytochrome
oxidase, of the fluoride anion on phosphoenolpyruvase, of fluoroace-
tates on aconitase, and of novobiocin on glucuronyltransferase to real-
ize the importance of this approach to toxicological evaluation. Enzyme inhibition may explain the toxic phenomena found in routine tests
in laboratory animals or in observations in man. It may also provide
a basis for forecasting toxic effects by indicating the first steps in the
process.

The difficulties are to select the right enzymes for study and the
most significant sites (body fluids, tissues, cells or subcellular fractions) for the measurement of changes in enzyme activity brought
about by the substance under test. This is probably why, in the field
of food additives, this approach has been so little used (105).

In conclusion, the effects of food additives on basic enzyme systems, as a part of biochemical and metabolic studies, may be expected
to contribute significantly to the understanding of the interrelationships
between the additive and other chemicals in the environment (106).

4.6 Acute Toxicity Studies

The phrase "acute toxicity test" implies the study of the effects produced by the test material when administered in a single dose. The
acute toxicity tests should give sufficient information to enable compari-
sons of the toxicity of related materials to be made and to provide the
necessary information for the planning of further studies. Acute toxicity
tests may indicate variation among species and yield some information
on the signs of intoxication and pathological effects.

It is advisable to employ at least three animal species, one of which
should be a non-rodent. Both sexes should be used in at least one spe-

cies. When doses greater than 5 g/kg of body-weight produce no deaths in the test animals an accurate determination of the lethal dose is unnecessary. With lethal doses under 5 g/kg body-weight the LD_{50} in one species should be determined by an appropriate method. For other species it is desirable to determine the approximate lethal dose, where this is less than 5 g/kg body-weight in order to indicate whether there is an important difference in species susceptibility.

The test material should be administered orally and parenterally. Where possible it should be administered as a solution in water, edible oil or other suitable solvent. If this is not possible an inert suspending agent may be used. In all cases control data should be available on any vehicle employed.

The animals should be observed for a period of 2 to 4 weeks, depending on their condition. Observation should include the onset, nature and duration of toxic signs, and mortality. It is important that autopsies be performed on some animals that die during the study and on some of the survivors once the study is completed. Microscopic examination of tissues should be carried out if the macroscopic study indicates that it is needed (107, 108).

4.7 Short-term Studies

These studies include all investigations other than those continued for most of the animal's life span. They are commonly carried out over 10% of the life span or less. As a rule, a number of different species are used. It is probable that the majority of toxic effects can be demonstrated in such studies (109, 110).

The dosage level at which deleterious effects occur, the time taken to cause them, and the nature of the effects produced are all of interest and potential importance. Relevant observations in man may be helpful in revealing gross species differences (109).

The purposes of the short-term test are to examine the biological nature of toxic effects, to assess possible cumulative action, to measure the variation in species sensitivity, to observe the nature of macro- and microscopic changes, and to determine the approximate dose level at which these effects occur. The test may yield information sufficient to show that the material is too toxic to warrant further study. It may also provide guidance for the selection of dosage for long-term tests and indicate special studies that may be necessary.

At least two species, including a rodent and a non-rodent, should be used. The number of animals should be large enough to allow for a statistical evaluation of the data. In the feeding experiments a sufficient number of levels should be selected to ensure that at least one level has no effect, and that doses are included which produce definite toxic effects, if possible. If no effects are observed at dosage levels of 10% in the diet, no useful purpose is served by employing higher levels. It is essential that a control group on the untreated diet be included in the experiment.

Observations should include general appearance, behavior, growth and mortality. In some cases estimation of food intake, studies of blood and urine chemistry and tests of organ functions may be indicated.

The study of the organs should include macroscopic and microscopic examination and measurement of the relative organ weights in the test and control groups (11, 104).

The above recommendations are still applicable except when the available data show that in the rat (often considered the animal of choice) the metabolism of the chemical being tested is not comparable with its metabolism in man.

It may be feasible or necessary to administer test substances by gavage or by capsule, e. g. , in cases of limited solubility, unpleasant taste, or need for accurate dosing. These procedures may produce effects different from those produced by adding a substance to the diet, either by increasing or decreasing the rate of absorption from the gastrointestinal tract or by influencing the metabolic pathway in the bacterial flora of the upper intestine. The validity of these forms of administration will depend on the substance tested (104).

4.8 Long-term Studies

Different opinions on different occasions have been expressed regarding long-term toxicity studies. Extensive description of long-term (chronic) toxicity studies appears in WHO/FAO reports. In these reports, the designation "long-term toxicity test" implies the study of the effects produced by the test material when administered in repeated doses over a longer period of time. Usually the major portion of the expected life span of short-lived species, sometimes covering the entire life span and more than one generation of such species.

Long-term toxicity tests are carried out to ascertain the maximum dosage level which produces no discernible ill-effects when administered over the major portion of the life span of the experimental animal, and to reveal effects which are not predictable from short-term tests.

In most cases the rat is the species of choice. Both sexes must be used. Under certain conditions the use of other species may be indicated.

A sufficient number of animals must be used in each experimental group to provide data for adequate statistical analysis. Consideration should be given to the expected mortality so that a sufficient number of survivors will be available for examination at the end of the experiment. This usually means that about 25 rats of each sex must be started on each level of dietary feeding. If the experiment is designed to involve the sacrifice of animals for pathological examination while it is in progress, additional animals in each group may be necessary.

In selecting the dosage levels to be fed, considerable information can be gained from the acute and especially from the short-term toxicity tests. In many cases, two dosage levels and a control of the basal diet without the additive are sufficient. The lowest dose should be so selected that animals receiving it throughout the experimental period will be expected to show no discernible ill-effects. On the other hand, the highest dosage level should, if possible, be such that a definite effect is produced by the test material. It should not, however, be so high that survival is markedly decreased. Dietary levels higher than

10% should not be used.

Dosage levels are commonly stated in terms of percentage of weight of the test material in the basal diet. However, dosage may be related to body-weight, body surface, or caloric intake to ensure uniformity of dosage throughout the experimental period and to facilitate comparison of data among species including man.

The mode of administration of choice is the oral route. However, in testing specifically for carcinogenicity it may be necessary to consider the advisability of parenteral administration.

It is customary to terminate long-term experiments on rats at the end of two years, since this is usually considered to cover the major portion of their life-span. However, it may often be desirable to terminate the experiments before this time--between 12 and 18 months--in order to avoid confusing signs of toxicity with the complicated pathological changes which occur in old animals. On the other hand, in special cases--where tumor formation is of primary concern--total life span studies, extending over two generations in at least one species, have been advocated and may be desirable.

In addition to other observations, attention should be given to effects on reproduction, lactation and offspring. Furthermore, it may be desirable to carry out macroscopic and microscopic examinations periodically during the course of the long-term test (112).

For reference (5) the most important tests in the category of chronic studies are those carried out over the greater part of the animal's life span. Such tests are essential for the assessment of the carcinogenic risk and they are also important for the evaluation of the acceptable level of a food additive, since it may be consumed daily for the whole life span. Long-term studies are almost always done in the rat, but with some food additives life span studies have also been done in the mouse (113).

For reference (6), long-term studies are those tests that have been carried out over the greater part of the animal's life span. Such tests are essential for assessing the carcinogenic risk. They are, generally speaking, the most important studies for the evaluation of the acceptable daily intakes of food additives, since these substances may be consumed by man for the whole life span. For the purpose of recording the data, a study is considered long-term if it has been carried out over one year in mice and rats or over five years in dogs (114).

The most recent opinion expressed on long-term toxicity studies asserts that where it is considered necessary to carry out long-term toxicity and carcinogenicity studies, the principles formulated in WHO Procedures (115) should be followed (116). (See Section 4.2.8 on the duration of toxicity tests in experimental animals.)

For a discussion on long-term studies for carcinogenicity testing see Section 4.9.3 on special studies which reports the opinions expressed in reference (64).

4.9 Special Studies

While this heading is rather confusing, it has been customary to include under it all investigations designed to detect a specific effect.

4.9.1 Reproduction, Embryotoxicity and Teratogenicity Studies

If during the course of short- or long-term studies or in a pilot experiment there is any evidence to suggest that reproduction may be affected, specific studies should be undertaken.

Reproduction studies must be carried out in a suitable species over at least two generations and may have to be continued over three or more. They should be designed to provide relevant information on fertility, progress of pregnancy, post-partum condition and progress of mothers and offspring.

Reproduction studies may be designed to include investigations on embryotoxicity and teratogenicity (116). By teratogenicity is meant a toxic effect on the embryo or fetus resulting in a congenital abnormality (117).

Alternatively it may be more convenient to conduct separate investigations on these aspects. Many suggested procedures for these studies have been published, but no one particular design has yet emerged as being universally acceptable (116).

In the area of teratogenicity testing, reference is made of a report from a WHO Scientific Group on principles for the testing of drugs for this effect (118) which contains recommendations to improve the predictive value of teratological testing of drugs. These recommendations relate mainly to the choice of suitable animal species, the range of doses to be used in the tests, and the mode of administration. Advice is given on various technical procedures, such as the breeding and handling of experimental animals, the removal of offspring and the examination of fetuses and post-natal animals.

4.9.2 Mutagenicity Studies

Mutagenic action of chemical agents represents a problem since, although exposure to chemicals in the external environment is increasing, there is little information on their possible mutagenic action. This problem cannot be ignored, since it represents one of the potential risks from chemical exposure. However, insofar as food additives are concerned, this possible risk must always be considered in the context of toxicological hazards in general, including the possible mutagenic effects of food itself. No specific tests are recommended for the assessment of mutagenic risk. However, some safeguard is provided by multigeneration studies while stressing the difficulties of extrapolating experimental data on mutagenicity of chemical obtained in bacterial systems, yeasts, or Drosophila to possible hazards of food additives in man. These special procedures commonly used to detect mutagenic activity cannot be recommended as part of the routine investigation of a food additive (119).

Reference is made to a report from a WHO Scientific Group on evaluation and testing of drugs for mutagenicity (120) where it is recommended that all drugs should be evaluated for possible mutagenic action to provide an indication of whether or not experimental studies in animals are needed. Priorities for testing are established and the various

methods available are reviewed. The report includes descriptions of
a number of procedures for detecting mutagenic effects in man, both
by studies in individuals and epidemiological studies, and population
monitoring. The interpretation of the dose-response relationship and
the problem of making benefit-risk assessments for drugs of known or
suspected mutagenic action used in the treatment of severe disease are
also discussed.

Many known mutagenic agents belong to classes of chemicals that
need metabolic activation. Lack of metabolic activation has been one
of the principal limitations of studies in in vitro and microbial systems.
Furthermore, the activation process in submammalian systems, e.g.
Drosophila, might be different from that in mammals and man. The
development of in vitro systems, including metabolic activation systems derived from mammals or man, may make possible rapid screening of substances. Data from such systems would be of value for setting priorities for more definitive mammalian testing (121).

Dealing with the assessment of the carcinogenicity and mutagenicity
of chemicals, the conclusion has been reached that in vitro mutagenicity tests alone cannot yield definitive results applicable to man, and
that mammalian test systems are more promising but still require
further development and experience.

No single test system can detect and characterize all mutagenic
agents. Therefore, the use of several tests is desirable and these
should primarily be done in mammals. In addition, a number of in
vitro and submammalian test systems might be used to answer specific question (122).

4.9.3 Carcinogenicity Studies

Testing procedures which would help in the evaluation of the carcinogenic hazards of food additives have been discussed on several occasions. Thus (1), it is stated that the occurrence of any tumors should
be given full attention. If more tumors are observed in the treated
animals than in the controls, or if a chemical relationship between the
additive under examination and known carcinogens exists, a special
study directed towards the evaluation of possible carcinogenic action
is indicated. Although such studies can be valuable for the detection of
carcinogenicity, there are unfortunately no completely satisfactory
methods available at this time for the evaluation of this hazard for
man. However, in the case of substances not clearly suspected of a
carcinogenic action on the basis of present knowledge, the life span
test suggested can be considered to be a reasonable safeguard against
the inclusion of a carcinogen as a food additive (123).

WHO/FAO reports discuss the whole problem of testing procedures
for carcinogenicity at length (64).

It is evident from a review of the literature that tests on experimental
animals cannot provide irrefutable proof of the safety from carcinogenicity of a substance for the human species. However, it is as least re-
assuring that the known carcinogenic activities of certain chemicals in
man are similar in many ways to those found in experimental animals.
Hence it is only prudent to determine, so far as it is practicable, the

carcinogenicity in experimental animals of substances used as food additives or occurring as contaminants. The results of such tests should determined to a considerable degree whether or not these substances should be used in the human diet. It is therefore necessary to formulate practical procedures for the determination of possible carcinogenicity within the limits of our present knowledge.

It is desirable that all food additives and contaminants be fully investigated. It must be recognized, however, that there are many substances which require study, and that some permitted lists contain apparently untested substances. It is also recognized that the available facilities and experienced personnel for carrying out such studies are limited and may remain so for an unpredictable time. Therefore, the proposed tests should be relatively simple and no more time consuming than necessary to facilitate the testing of as many food additives as possible within a reasonable period of time.

It has been emphasized that the details of tests of food additives for the potential carcinogenicity are the responsibility of the interested scientist (124). Nevertheless, some general and special recommendations may be given to make the investigations as informative as possible and acceptable internationally (125).

Several factors must be taken into account in deciding the scope of the tests required in the case of any particular substance--namely, the nature of the substance, impurities present, the proposed use, the particular food involved, the amount which is likely to be eaten, and the age and physical condition of the main consumers. Such considerations would allow for reasonable priorities in testing to be established and thus provide broader safeguards in the shortest possible time (125).

The view has been adopted that the minimum safeguard must be an investigation of the tumor incidence in a chronic toxicity test as set forth in general terms (126). This should involve the study of an adequate number of animals of two species (e.g., rats and mice) subjected to the feeding of a suitable dose range of the substance under question for the lifetime of the animals. Where additional safeguards are considered necessary, because of the nature of the food additive or of its proposed use, further tests, such as the use of a suitable parenteral route of administration or studies in other species of animal, are recommended (125).

More recently, the relationship between mutagenesis and carcinogenesis was discussed (3). Current theories postulate similarities between the mechanisms of mutagenesis and the mode of action of major groups of chemical and physical carcinogens.

There is increasing evidence that many chemical carcinogens in their carcinogenically reactive form can induce mutations in microbial and some mammalian test systems. But it is impossible to assess whether or not these common properties of many chemical carcinogens and mutagens also point to common sequences of events resulting in a cancer cell or a mutated cell. Furthermore, some potent mutagens do not appear to be carcinogenic in any of the test systems used and certain carcinogens have not been demonstrated to be mutagenic. One major difficulty in the comparison of mutagenic and carcinogenic actions is the use of results obtained from different test systems. Induction of point mutations is reported mostly from studies in microbial systems, whereas chromosomal abnormalities have been observed in tissue culture and, more recently, in vivo studies in rodents. A second difficulty arises from the need for metabolic activation of many chemical mutagens and carcinogens. Until recently most in vitro systems used in mutagenesis bioassay have lacked this activation potential. It is thought that metabolic activation converting a precarcinogen into the "ultimate" carcinogen is analogous to the change from a premutagen to the ultimate mutagen (127).

It was concluded that the relationship between carcinogenesis and mutagenesis requires further investigation. However, the association between mutagenicity and carcinogenicity of many compounds is sufficiently great to justify the use of mutagenicity tests as prescreening procedures for possible carcinogens (122).

Furthermore, the in vitro test systems using cell transformation in tissue culture as an end point hold promise as a substitute test for the animal carcinogen bioassay.

Other test systems make use of the capacity of some, if not all, reactive forms of chemical carcinogens to interact with DNA. Mutagenicity tests may have value as a prescreening procedure for carcinogenicity. However, for the time being, the histologic verification of tumor development in the whole animal must be the ultimate test for carcinogenic activity (128).

In testing food additives for carcinogenic action, certain aspects need particular careful consideration. For example, a promoting effect detected in the course of a carcinogenicity test cannot be ignored. However, routine testing for promoting effects should not be used until more is known about its mechanism and how broadly it can be applied. Likewise, even when cancer is produced by chemicals administered by other than the oral route, their evaluation for food additive use requires experiments using oral administration.

Tissue culture methods for the study of neoplastic transformation using chemical carcinogens have not yet been fully developed, and it would be premature to introduce these methods into toxicity studies of food additives.

A procedure at present under investigation in routine carcinogenesis studies includes the use of two parent and offspring generations to take into account the transplacental transport of carcinogens and their transfer to milk. No recommendation can yet be made as to the suitability of this method for the toxicological investigation of food additives (129).

In the context of carcinogenicity testing reference should be also made to a report (130) on principles for testing and evaluation of drugs for carcinogenic hazards, a distinction being drawn between testing a drug for carcinogenicity in animals and evaluating its carcinogenic hazard to man. Criteria are proposed for deciding the stage of experimental and clinical development at which drugs should be tested. Detailed recommendations are given for testing drugs in animals, and brief reference is made to retrospective and prospective studies in man. Guidelines for the pathological examination of experimental animals are also provided.

4.10 Observations in Man

The subject of investigations in human beings has been approached on several occasions. It has been recognized that observations in man are of prime importance because of the differences between one species and another in reactions to toxic substances and the subsequent uncertainty when extrapolating data from animals experiments to human beings.

Studies in man may be carried out by the careful observation of individuals who have ingested the test compound. Additional data may be obtained by studying individuals exposed to additives occupationally or who have come in contact with them through accidental ingestion. Finally, studies may also be carried out in populations consuming a given additive at high levels because of ethnic proclivities for therapeutic purposes (129).

The usefulness of these studies, coupled with results obtained in experimental animals for predictive purposes, has also been emphasized. Studies in experimental animals on the biological effects of chemicals that may be introduced into the environment have the prediction of any possible hazard to man as one of their major objectives. One of the greatest problems that arises in these studies is in the extrapolation of the data obtained from investigations in animals and to the definition of safe levels of exposure in man. The purpose for which the chemical may eventually be used does not necessarily affect the nature of the investigational problems involved.

The prediction and prevention of possible toxic hazards to the community that might arise from the introduction of a chemical into the environment can be made more certain if information from meaningful studies in human subjects is available. Three particular aspects of toxicology require consideration in this connexion: first, the choice of the most appropriate animal species for investigations that aim at the prediction of human responses; secondly, the investigation of a reversible specific effect observed in the most sensitive animal species to determine whether it represents a significant hazard to man; and thirdly, the study of effects specific to man (131).

In the case of drugs, the effects specific to man may be revealed during clinical trials or as a result of the reporting of adverse reactions after the drug is placed on the market.

In the case of other chemicals, it is not acceptable to study such effects by the use of volunteers. Toxicological studies can be made in those who are occupationally exposed to the chemical or in patients suffering from accidental poisoning. There is a need for more critical epidemiological and toxicological investigations in such situations. If unexpected effects apparently specific to man are observed, it is advisable to re-examine the evidence obtained earlier from animal studies to determine whether useful information in those investigations was missed or whether some different method of study might have been of greater predictive value.

Ethical and legal problems may arise in connection with the provision of volunteers for these investigations. Since the situation differs greatly from country to country, it should be left to the appropriate authorities in each country to decide any issues involved (132).

Studies in human volunteers are useful for confirming predicted safety margin. Chemicals intended for use as drugs are subjected to human pharmacological investigations and to clinical trials that must, of necessity, involve the use of biologically effective dosage levels. In the examination of other chemicals from a toxicological point of view, it is sometimes necessary to ascertain whether the safety margin predicted from animal data is valid. For this purpose it may be helpful to administer the chemical to human volunteers. It is emphasized that the following conditions should be fulfilled with regard to such a study:

a. The chemical should have been fully studied in a range of experimental animals.
b. There should be a clear need, in the public interest, for the study of some effect or effects in the human subject.
c. The effect or effects studied should be reversible.
d. The dose levels used should be based on full information of the toxicological properties of the substance in animals.
e. The investigation should be terminated immediately once the effect has been unequivocally demonstrated (132).

The importance of these recommendations with regard to the desirability of supplementing animal studies on additives by investigations in man was considered to apply especially to additives to be used in infant food (133). Biochemical studies in human subjects should be encouraged. In this regard it has been observed that one aspect of metabolic studies that has not received enough attention so far is the study of the metabolic pathways in man. Although this presents considerable difficulties, information on the main pathways of metabolism in man might be helpful in choosing the most appropriate animal for long-term studies. There are often quite marked differences in metabolism between animal species. If a choice of experimental animal for long-term studies of a substance is made without knowing in which species (if any) the metabolism of the substance is substantially similar to that in man, there is a danger that the choice may not be an inappropriate one and the results of the studies consequently may be of little relevance to the problem of assessing the human hazard involved in the use of the substance as a food additive. It may be noted, however, that the paucity of information on metabolism in man has been taken into account in assessing the acceptable intakes. The rates of metabolism and elimination are also important, since they give an indication of the likelihood of accumulation. In general, cumulative substances must be considered unsuitable for use as food additives (134).

There is a need at a relatively early stage to obtain information on the absorption, distribution, metabolism and elimination of the chemical in human subjects. This makes it possible to compare this information with that obtained in various animal species and to choose the species that is most likely to have a high predictive value for human responses.

The sooner these studies at a low dosage level can be undertaken in the course of toxicological investigation, the better. However, it is

necessary to have adequate short-term toxicological information in
several species before even low doses of a new chemical are administered to human subjects (137).

Therefore it is desirable, and in many cases necessary, to study
the metabolic fate and effects of food additives in man. Such investigations, which should be carefully planned and controlled, form a valuable part of the evaluation of safety (88).

The problem that arises in connection with early human studies in
the investigation of drug toxicity is discussed by WHO (136). In this
report methods of safety testing are reviewed under two main headings:
biochemical studies and pharmacological and toxicological studies. The
biochemical studies discussed include absorption, distribution, excretion and metabolism of a drug, since knowledge of these factors controlling drug action is of fundamental importance for proper evaluation of
toxicity. Recognized procedures for pharmacological and toxicological
studies are also described, and attention is paid to the timing and nature of first studies in man.

4.11 Unconventional Studies

Toxicological data obtained from experiments using unconventional
methods may provide useful background information and, while of
little prospective use, may contribute in retrospect to the understanding of toxic effects (137). These are studies in which non-oral routes
of administration, the use of an unusual species, or unconventional
procedures not of direct value in making toxicological assessments
are used.

The need to expose experimental animals in a way that parallels
human exposure has been discussed in a similar context when the
toxicity of pesticide residues in food were considered (138, 139). Rats
normally feed more or less continuously during the night. When such
species are used for testing substances that act only briefly and do
not accumulate or produce cumulative effects, it is to be expected that
dietary administration will cause less pronounced biological effects
than administration by gavage which permits the total daily intake to
enter the body in a single dose. In almost every instance administration by gavage produces higher peak levels in blood and tissue than
does incorporation in the diet. Experimental data from studies where
animals are fed a chemical as part of the feed show obvious differences
from data obtained in experiments where the compound is administered
by gavage. Therefore experiments using gavage cannot replace feeding
experiments for testing of materials found or suspected of being found
in food.

An opinion was also expressed regarding short-term screening tests
being developed which will enable large numbers of substances including
food additives and food contaminants to be screened rapidly and economically for carcinogenicity and other manifestations of toxicity. The
interpretation of the results of these rapid tests in terms of likely
hazard to man is at present not clearly defined when compared with
the results obtained from the generally accepted testing procedures.

Such tests might eventually be added to the conventional approach used in screening and setting priorities for complete toxicological evaluations of various compounds (140).

5. CONSIDERATIONS ON PRINCIPLES OF INTERPRETATION OF EXPERIMENTAL FINDINGS

5.1. Responsibility

As the conduct of the experiment designed to test safe use of food additives is the responsibility of the scientist, so also is the evaluation and interpretation of the data from these experiments. In order that sound decisions can be made regarding the use of food additives, the scientific data that have been assembled must be made available in a form that will allow independent scientists with the appropriate experience to make an adequate assessment of the findings. The decisions reached by expert groups in different countries with respect to any particular food additive may vary, since the relative importance of different aspects of the problem may be affected by the circumstances, dietary habits or legislative background of the community that the expert group serves (141).

5.2 Acute and Conventional-approach Studies

An assessment of acute toxicity is often used to give an indication of the usefulness of a food additive. Clearly a satisfactory food additive is likely to be a substance of low acute toxicity. A substance that shows appreciable acute toxicity should be regarded with suspicion until its safety under conditions of use has been demonstrated by further studies.

Frequently, owing to the low toxicity of the test material, it is only possible to state that the LD_{50} exceeds 5 g/kg body-weight. The main value of the acute tests in such cases is to provide information on the effects of the test material on biological systems. These observations are of great importance since they may indicate the further studies needed.

Acute toxicity tests should provide information on species specificity. The objective is to reduce the possibility that some important effect that might occur in man is being overlooked in the main test animal (142).

Data on acute toxicity is usually of limited value in the evaluation of the toxicological risk of a food additive. However, the LD_{50} gives some indication of the general toxicity class and the difference between the oral and the parenteral LD_{50} levels may sometimes be of interest. The studies are usually performed on several species, and this may give some indication of species differences (143, 144).

Studies on acute toxicity in several animal species should make it possible to gain an idea of the apparent mode of action of the chemical-- e.g., whether it acts as an anticholineasterase, central nervous system depressant or convulsant, a metabolic stimulant, or a liver- or kidney-damaging agent.

Comparison with well known chemicals may be useful when a new chemical falls into the same general category (145). For a number of flavoring substances the data for acute oral toxicity suggested that little absorption occurred by this route. In such cases, information on acute toxicity following intraperitoneal administration could give a guide to the toxic potential of the substance. A short description of the toxic signs and an indication of the time and cause of death would be useful when reporting such studies (146).

Short-term and long-term studies should provide data on the cumulative effects of the test material (147).

5.3 Decrease in Rate of Body-weight Gain

Changes in normal body-weight activity may be brought about by many factors such as an alteration of water intake, increased water loss, an alteration of food or calorie intake or faulty utilization of absorbed nutrients. These various effects may be due to a toxic action of the substance under investigation or to causes that are not relevant to the assessment of toxic potential. Diarrhea due to an osmotic effect at high dosage levels of the test substance, or the interference with the palatability of the diet by the presence of the test substance are but two examples. The effects that are irrelevant to toxicity should be differentiated from true toxic effects by appropriate studies. A decrease in the rate of body-weight gain, accompanied by a corresponding reduction of food intake, should not be assumed to be caused by a palatability defect, since the reduction of food intake may be due to toxic anorexia. If a palatability defect is present, this may be disclosed by a preference test in which the diets fed to the control and experimental groups are compared (151).

The observation of decreased rate of body-weight gain requires further study to differentiate between toxicologically relevant and irrelevant effects. A preference test may distinguish between palatability defect and toxic anorexia (148, 146).

5.4 Liver Enlargement

The occurrence of liver enlargement in the absence of other apparent changes in this organ has often been reported in toxicological studies. Customarily, hepatomegaly has been considered to indicate a pathological change, and this interpretation has been applied in establishing "no-effect" levels. It is reasonable to believe that this alteration may not always represent a pathological change and in some instances may, on investigation, be revealed to be a normal response to an increased work load. This seemingly logical contention requires substantiation. It is recommended that detailed investigation of liver enlargement in toxicity tests be carried out (as set out below), including a study not only of the absolute weight of the liver (measured under standard conditions) but also of the relationship of the weight of the liver to body-weight, provided that the growth and condition of the animals justifies the calculation of the relative liver weight on this basis. If this is not the case, for example because of emaciation, liver weight may be related to the weight of the heart or brain for purposes of comparison with control groups.

In studies on food additives it is usual to administer the substance under investigation at several dose levels. At least some of these are far in excess of those that are ever likely to be administered to man. Such high dose levels of a metabolizable chemical substance must inevitably increase the load on the liver, if this organ plays any part in its metabolism. It is known that under these circumstances the endoplasmic reticulum in the liver cells frequently proliferates, elaborating more enzymes and thereby facilitating the metabolism of the compound. It is likely, therefore, that liver enlargement will often be observed in animal studies on the biological effects of new substances proposed for use as food additives.

To evaluate fully the significance of such findings the following studies are recommended:

a. Liver morphology; ultrastructural studies;
b. Detailed investigation of the relationship to the dose and to the time of development of hepatomegaly during feeding experiments;
c. Reversibility of liver enlargement on continuing dosage and on cessation of administration of the compound;
d. Additional criteria of liver response and the relationship of these to dose and liver enlargement. Such criteria may include the activities of microsomal-processing (drug-metabolizing) enzymes in the liver and of glucose-6-phosphatase or other indicators of changes taking place within the liver in response to exposure to the test compound (149, 152).

5.5 Enzymes in the Blood and in Tissues

An increase in the level of certain enzymes in the blood may be indicative of tissue damage. From this point of view, transaminases and other intracellular enzymes have been studied. When tissue damage occurs, these enzymes may leak out of the cells and cause a significant increase in blood enzyme levels. Such changes have been extensively studied in clinical biochemical laboratories in relation to myocardial damage following infarction and, in this instance, the time relationships between the occurrence of myocardial damage and alterations in the blood enzyme levels are important. Alterations in glutamic-pyruvic transaminase and glutamic-oxaloacetic transaminase have been observed to follow liver damage. Damage to a number of other organs has also been associated with various changes in blood enzyme levels. Changes of this sort may be useful in indicating that tissue damage is caused gradually, enzymes may be lost from the tissue cells without causing a demonstrable change in blood enzyme levels.

Some food additives produce their effects by enzyme inhibition. Thus, in molds, sorbic acid inhibits a number of enzymes, including catalase and alcohol dehydrogenase, and its fungistatic properties are probably related to this effect. However, in the animal body, metabolic degradation makes it impossible to administer enough sorbic acid by mouth to cause significant inhibition of dehydrogenase systems. Study of the effect of food additives on enzymes should be encouraged.

Apart from enzyme inhibition, the level of tissue enzymes may also give some indication of toxicity. As already mentioned, when cells are damaged, intracellular enzymes may enter the blood. The level of these released enzymes in the blood depends on the relative rates at which the enzymes leave the cell and are inactivated or otherwise eliminated. The acuteness and severity of the damage and the timing of changes in relation to damage are significant factors in determining the blood level Loss from the tissues will lead to a diminished enzyme concentration in the cell, unless regeneration keeps pace with the rate of loss. Thus, the cellular enzymes may indicate either acute or chronic damage and measurement of these levels might prove useful in the differentiation of toxic and toxicologically irrelevant changes in cells and organs.

Another aspect of enzyme changes of toxicological interest is the induction of so-called drug-metabolizing enzymes, especially in the liver. Some substances cause a considerable increase in many of these enzymes, which are found in the microsomal fraction of liver cells. This increase enables the animal to metabolize greater amounts of the substrate and other substances. The products of metabolism may be more or less toxic than the original substance. If the products are less toxic, the tolerance of the animal to the original substance may greatly increase. However, not all substances induce metabolizing enzymes, and some may take several weeks before causing significant induction. Examples of the former are parathion and isopropanol and of the latter are carbaryl and, to a less extent, methoxychlor and TDI (2, 2,-Bis (p-chlorophenyl)-1, 1-dichloroethane) (150). These biochemical changes may or may not be related to ultrastructural changes in hepatic cells. They are often quickly reversible and may represent adaptation of the cell to the administered chemical.

Investigation of these phenomena as a part of the biochemical and metabolic studies may be expected to contribute significantly to the understanding of the interrelationships between the additive and other chemicals in the environment (153).

Cholinesterases in both plasma and erythrocytes are markedly reduced by a number of substances. There is, however, poor correlation between the cholinesterase levels and the signs and symptoms of toxicity. Blood cholinesterase levels may be useful as an indication of exposure to a substance with anticholinesterase activity, but not as an invariable guide to the degree of intoxication present or predicted. In general, lack of a chemical or one of its metabolites, at some specified site (for example, in blood) and the occurrence of toxic signs or symptoms may be due to the fact that the more significant change in activity or concentration is occurring at some other site (for example, at nerve endings). Thus, the changes being measured may correlate with changes at the more significant site only over a small part of the range. Alternatively, some other enzyme, chemical, or metabolite may be more closely related to the toxic mechanism. Although changes in blood cholinesterase levels may be helpful in toxicological studies, it is important that further research should be done to relate the indices used as closely as possible to the biochemical changes concerned in bringing about the toxic effects. In this context, special attention should be paid to the method of estimating cholinesterases (154).

5.6 Impurities or Transformation Products

The relationship between chemical and biological reactivity of a food additive should not be assumed but must be demonstrated. Thus, the suggestion which has been sometimes made that because a food additive is chemically inert in would be without long-term toxic effects is not valid. There is sufficient experimental evidence to demonstrate that such assumptions are not always valid and therefore adequate toxicological studies are always indispensable.

Toxic metabolites may be formed by the intestinal microflora. The formation of cyclohexylamine from cyclamate examplifies the possibility of the generation of toxic metabolites from food additives. In this and other instances, the microflora of the alimentary tracts of man and of the animal species used in toxicological testing behave similarly. However, it is possible that the different micro-organisms colonizing human and animal intestinal tracts could generate different toxic metabolites from the same food additive.

The information of toxic products by interaction between an additive and a food constituent should also be considered. If such a reaction product can be identified, then it can be subjected to appropriate toxicological investigation and the results can be evaluated. Furthermore, it is possible that unidentified toxic products may be formed. In this case, foodstuffs treated with the additive should be used in experiments (156).

Impurities or transformation products that are more toxic than the parent food additive are illustrated by the following examples. The presence of up to 6 g of ortho-toluenesulfonamide per kilogram of saccharin has been reported and may have been the cause of the magnesium ammonium phosphate calculi that occurred in rats fed very high doses of saccharin. Ethylurethane is formed in amounts of the order of 0.01-0.04 mg/litre in beverages treated with diethylpyrocarbonate, depending on the pH and ammonium content. The transformation of nitrates to nitrites in food or water or in the gastrointestinal tract of young infants, as well as the possibility of the formation of nitroso compounds, is made largely by interaction with secondary and tertiary amines. Cyclohexylamine may occur as a manufacturing impurity in cyclamate, but much larger amounts of cyclohexylamine may be formed by the action on cyclamate of anaerobic bacteria in the gut (48).

5.7 Mutagenicity

The significance of results of mutagenicity studies on food additives cannot yet be interpreted in terms of human health hazards (155). In vitro mutagenicity tests alone cannot yield definite results applicable to man. Mammalian test systems are more promising but still require further development and experience. However, the possible existence of a threshold to the effects of chemical mutagens should be envisaged (156).

5.8 Carcinogenicity

5.8.1 The Problem of Interpreting Results

The interpretation of the results of test procedures in experimental carcinogenesis can be divided into two parts:

    a. The consideration of the accuracy and significance of the experimental studies;
    b. The evaluation of these facts, as well as epidemiological evidence, in terms of the carcinogenic risk in man.

When the risk has been estimated, appropriate action must be decided upon on the merits of each case (157).

5.8.2 Considerations of Experimental Procedures

Design of the experiment: There are examples in the literature of attempts to interpret and evaluate unsatisfactory experimental work. It cannot be too strongly emphasized that the wide knowledge and experience needed for these investigations are required from the start. No amount of subsequent pathological interpretation or statistical analysis will extract sound information from poorly planned or executed experiments. First attention should be given to the quality of the work presented. The publication of experimental studies of poor quality and interpretation can only raise an ill-founded suspicion that a possible carcinogenic risk may exist.

If such an investigation gives rise to a doubt about the safety of a substance that may occur infood, it is clearly in the public interest that further work be done. If, however, the evidence is not adequate to form a sound opinion, it would be wiser not to publish the information until adequate experimental evidence can be presented (158).

Material tested: The following are suggestions with regard to the information desired in publications of experimental studies in carcinogenesis:

    a. Identity, purity, physical and chemical properties of the substances tested and of the solvents or vehicles used;
    b. Concentration of the material under investigation in the wet or dry diet or in the solvent or in the vehicle used;
    c. If a positive control is used, precise information on any carcinogen used.

Animals under experimentation: The following are suggestions regarding animals used as subjects in carcenogenic investigation studies:

    a. Source, species, strain, sex, age, state of health and type of housing;

    b. Composition of the diet and, if appropriate, reasons for its choice;

    c. Number of animals at the beginning of experiment;

    d. Details and method of dosage;

    e. Conditions and routes of administration.

Observations of both experimental and control groups: The following information should be recorded carefully during the experimental period in order that the validity of the research can be substantiated beyound doubt:

    a. State of health of the animal;

    b. Average amount of food consumed;

    c. Survival times of all animals and time at which 50% of the animals were dead;

    d. Time at which toxic effects and/or tumor production were noted;

    e. Post-mortem findings;

    f. Number, sites and histological nature of any tumors observed. (159).

5.8.3 Pathology

Since the assessment of tumor incidence is the crux of the evaluation of the carcinogenic risk, it is of great importance that all the animals should be subjected to adequate autopsy and histopathological examination. In many countries there appears to be a need for more people adequately trained in the pathology of laboratory animals.

Exact descriptions and precise diagnosis of tumors, as well as proper differentiation of neoplastic and non-neoplastic lesions, is not a unique need of investigations concerned with the possible carcinogenic hazard from food additives. As in other fields of medicine, clinical and experimental, it is imperative that the diagnoses be exact and clear. Otherwise, faulty interpretation of food additive studies and practical decisions based upon them, may result.

Chemical substances or other agents continuously fed or introduced into the body by some other route might result in a variety of toxic and/or neoplastic manifestations in tissues and organs--for example, vascular disturbance, degeneration, acute or chronic inflammation, hyperplasia, metaplasia, and benign and malignant neoplasms. These manifestations must be recognized, described, differentiated and classified. Vague and inexact descriptions and nomenclature such as "lesion," "pathologic change," "alteration," "tumor" or "cancer" are inadequate and confusing. More importantly, they may lead to unacceptable evaluation and dangerous or unfair practical decisions.

For example, what are the various lesions that might possibly occur in the liver through the action of a chemical or other agent incorporated into the diet? Some of these actually encountered in practice are various types of degeneration: dilatation of the sinusoids, in aggravated form appearing as blood cysts; acute inflammations; chronic inflammations and fibrosis (cirrhosis); cholangiofibrosis, sometimes mistaken for neoplasms; hyperplastic nodules of liver parenchyma (regeneration nodules), sometimes mistaken for benign hepatomas; and of course neoplasms such as benign hepatomas, cholangiocarcinomas and hepatocellular carcinomas. Obviously, precise recognition of pathological findings is only one of the factors in experimental design, execution and evaluation, but without it the others may lose importance and significance.

In the assessment of the carcinogenic risk it is not considered relevant whether the tumor is benign or malignant since the conversion of the first to the second must be regarded as possible (160).

5.8.4 Routes of Administration and Local Sarcomas

It is imperative that the carcinogenic risk of a food additive or contaminant be tested by the means or route involved in its actual use-- that is, ingestion. The question arises as to whether other routes of administration of the chemical substance or agent--such as subcutaneous or intraperitoneal injection, or application to the skin--might provide additional information or proof of its potential carcinogenicity. Should this property be definitely established through feeding experiments, no need exists for investigations concerned with other routes of administration.

Suppose, however, that the results of adequate feeding studies reveal no carcinogenicity. It has been suggested that the safety of the agent should be further studied by injecting the material into the subcutaneous tissue of experimental animals. This procedure is practised by some investigators. In some instances, this procedure has resulted in the production of a high incidence of local sarcomas without inducing the formation of neoplasms in other tissues.

What is the biological significance of the results of such a series of experiments in relation to the problem of food additives? As the two-route studies have been described, it is obvious that the induction of local sarcomas is not a proof that the agent will be carcinogenic on feeding. However, such divergent findings are less satisfactory that those where the agent is non-carcinogenic by both routes or by others that might be employed. Repetition and extension of the investigations might reveal evidence helpful in reaching a sound decision. The contradictory results of the feeding and injection studies might suggest the need for searching for a possible alternative substance which gives less reason for concern. For example, in some countries it is recommended that colors which produce local sarcomas when injected should be replaced by others, if functionally equivalent, which do not produce any significant tumor increase in animal experimentation by any route of administration.

Why does the induction of sarcomas, in the absence of carcinogenesis on feeding, leave uncertainty as to the value of the former findings? It is known that local sarcomas may be induced by chemical carcinogens, by some in minute amounts. However, certain plastics, metals, and glass, when placed subcutaneously in sheet or plate form, have also been demonstrated to result in sarcomas. Their activity appears to be related to physical form. The possibility exists that certain other chemical substances may induce sarcomas by this latter mechanism, yet reveal no activity in exhaustive ingestion studies. Nevertheless it has been ruled out that such substances may induce local sarcomas on the basis of their chemical reactivity. This is the status of our present knowledge, on which practical decisions must be made. Because of the absence of definite proof, decisions with regard to inclusion in permitted lists of substances giving rise only to local sarcomas at the injection site differ from country to country. This is unsatisfactory and clearly shows that in this area, as in others related to the food additive problem, more research is needed (161).

Results of new developments since these views were presented determined the following recommendations with regard to the significance of the occurrence of sarcomas following subcutaneous injections. It is recommended:

a. That for the routine testing of food additives and contaminants, the subcutaneous injection test should be considered inappropriate unless special conditions, such as lack of absorption from the gastrointestinal tract under conditions of routine feeding to experimental animals, demand additional studies;

b. that the occurrence of local sarcoma following subcutaneous injection of food additives or contaminants should not, alone, be considered significant evidence of a carcinogenic hazard. Such a finding, however, indicates the desirability of a thorough study for systemic manifestations of carcinogenicity by other parenteral or further specific oral investigations (162).

5.8.5 Dietary Considerations

The genesis of neoplasms is influenced, in varying degrees, by the dietary and nutritional state of the host. Chronic caloric restriction strikingly inhibits the formation of many types of tumor. This effect has been demonstrated for all varieties of tumors investigated. Conversely, fat-enrichment of the diet augments the formation of certain tumors, but has no effect on others. As a generality, modifications of the dietary levels of protein, vitamins and minerals have lesser effects.

It is worth noting at least two important exceptions to this generality. A number of investigators have shown that high levels of dietary riboflavin retard the genesis of liver neoplasms in rats fed 4-dimethyl-aminoazobenzene, regardless of the general nature of the diet. On the other hand, some strains of rat having a high requirement for choline develop liver tumors when chronically fed a choline-deficient ration.

The inhibitory influence of caloric restriction and lower body-weight may have direct implications in investigations on food additives. Restriction of calories or deprivation of essential components of the diet may be a part of an experiment, but can occur also without the intention or knowledge of the investigator. For example, animals subjected to various agents (hormones, anti-metabolites, carcinogens, other chemicals--including the substance under investigation--or irradiation) may reduce their food intake or develop an increased need for particular dietary essentials. Intercurrent infections can cause diarrhea or loss of appetite. These and other circumstances could bring on subnormal food consumption, altered metabolism, lower body-weight and a shortened life span. Should any of these conditions become a factor in an experiment, the genesis of expected tumors might be retarded--and possible induced neoplasms might not be evoked. Caloric restriction and low body-weight are not the common denominators of all inhibitory effects, but for more exact interpretation the nutritional status of the animals should be known.

Conversely, the addition to the diet of a lipid material or mixture or of a substance dissolved in a lipid medium may result in the potentiation or augmentation of carcinogenesis. If the experimental animal under study has a normal expectancy of a small incidence of one or more types of neoplasms, addition of lipids to the diet may result in a higher incidence at an earlier average time of appearance. This cannot be interpreted as induction of tumors by a carcinogen.

It can be seen from this brief consideration of dietary factors that the general condition and nutritional state of the experimental animal, as well as the specific influence of a particular additive on its dietary intake and metabolism, may play a significant role in the production of neoplasms (86).

5.8.6 Threshold

On the subject of substance concentration it is of interest to compare some statements. A WHO evaluation report (64) states that the presence of carcinogenic substances in food might be a significant factor in the occurrence of what is considered to be spontaneous cancer in man and animals. Since dose response relationships have been demonstrated in the case of carcinogenic agents, the reduction of carcinogenic substances in food to the lowest practicable level may be one of the effective measures towards cancer prevention. Many factors may influence dose-response in carcinogenesis. Their complexities are such that it is agreed that no assuredly safe level for carcinogens in human food can be determined from experimental findings at the present time and that the elimination, or at least reduction to a minimum, of all proved carcinogenic substances in the diet of man and of animals used as human food is a worthwhile objective (163).

A WHO assessment study (3) states the following findings: (a) it is recognized that there are certain instances of cancer induction that may be secondary to an initial noncarcinogenic effect of a chemical; (b) the role of modifying factors, enhancing or inhibiting the effect of carcinogens, must be considered; (c) assessment of risk must involve a knowledge of the environmental "background" levels of the chemicals concerned; (d) newer knowledge of DNA repair mechanisms and of immunological influences may have a bearing on the evaluation of the effects of low doses of chemical carcinogens; and (e) that the possible existence of a threshold to the effects of both chemical carcinogens and mutagens should be envisaged (164).

In this same assessment paper (3) the concept of threshold for carcinogens is further developed. For most biological effects it is assumed from experience that a threshold and a no-effect level exist. Threshold dose levels in mutagenesis have been questioned on the basis of studies of radiation-induced mutations and because mutations may even result from a change in only one base pair in DNA. For carcinogenesis the existence of a threshold has also been questioned because of:

a. The self-replicating nature of the cancer cell;
b. The work of Druckrey and others, which has been interpreted to indicate summation of irreversible effects in carcinogenesis (this has been expressed by Druckrey in the equation $Dt^n = k^3$, where n is greater than 1);
c. Evidence from experiments on tumor initiation and promotion in skin carcinogenesis indicating lasting change induced by one tumor-initiating event;
d. The fact that cancer can occur in response to chemicals, even after single doses, long after their disappearance from the body;
e. The possibility that cancer may result from mutation in a somatic cell.

The summation effect described by Druckrey and others is not questioned and his equation characterizing carcinogenic potency may be accepted. Nevertheless, every organism has a limited life span and in this sense there is, for each individual, a real threshold. Cigarette smoking is well known to cause human cancer in a dose-related fashion. The demonstration of a decline in the risk of developing lung cancer in ex-smokers means that these effects are partly reversible. Recent work on the initiation and promotion of tumors, in which application of the promoting agent was delayed for a longer time than in the earlier experiments, suggests that the effect of an initiating event may disappear, but this requires confirmation.

Knowledge of molecular biology has developed rapidly and it is now known that there are cellular mechanisms for the repair of DNA. These processes include single-strand and double-strand repair by excision or post-replication mechanisms. Most knowledge of DNA repair has come from investigations of microbial systems, but there are reasons to believe that similar processes occur in mammalian cells.

The repair of DNA usually shows exact fidelity but does not always lead to a perfect copy of the original DNA. Improper repair may result in the death or mutation of cells. Deleterious effects are more common after more severe DNA injury and when there is reduced capacity for repair. Impaired efficiency of repair may be genetically determined--e. g., in human subjects with the repair-deficient type of xeroderma pigmentosum. Several agents are known to interfere with DNA repair in microbial or mammalian cells in vitro.

In biological systems with an efficient DNA repair mechanism, the implication of an exposure threshold for point mutations and deletions is very strong. However, it is not established if such mechanisms are effectively present in various types of mammalian cells or if these mechanisms function in vivo. If cancer results from such mutations in a somatic cell, the above conclusions regarding a threshold may apply to carcinogenesis.

A number of chemically induced tumors possess antigenic properties capable of inducing immunological tumor-associated rejection
reactions. The existence of immunological surveillance mechanisms
that protect the host against neoplastic cells has been postulated. This
is supported by studies on host immunity to autochthonous tumors in
man and others. Immunodeficiency diseases lead to an increased risk
of neoplastic disease.

The degree of importance of tumor-limiting responses remains to
be analyzed qualitatively and quantitatively. The dichotomy of the
immune response--with mechanisms that both limit and facilitate
neoplastic growth--should be kept in mind.

Further basic studies are needed before a correlation between
chemical carcinogenesis and host immunity in man can be established.

From these considerations the existence of a threshold may be envisaged. Nevertheless the difficulties of determining a threshold for
a population are great. Therefore, mathematically derived conclusions
that it is impossible to demonstrate no-effect levels experimentally
cannot be ignored (165).

6. THE PROCESS OF EVALUATION AND
TOXICOLOGICAL DECISIONS (166)

6.1 General Observations

There are two stages in the toxicological evaluation of a substance
proposed for use as a food additive. The first is the collection of relevant data, which are usually derived from experimental testing in
laboratory animals and, whenever possible, from observations in man.
The second is the interpretation and assessment of the data in order
to arrive at a decision about the acceptability or rejection of the substance as a food additive.

The place of toxicological decisions in the assessment of food additives is indicated in Fig 1 which shows the flow of the process. The
diagram reported in the figure may be interpreted as follows: the
TOXICOLOGICAL METHODOLOGY 1 leads to the design of APPRO-
PRIATE INVESTIGATIONS 2 which ought to supply ADEQUATE IN-
FORMATION 3 which, after proper INTERPRETATION 4 could assist
in the formulation of TOXICOLOGICAL DECISIONS 5 which should
provide reasonable basis for REGULATIONS 6 on the safe use of intentional and unintentional food additives. Steps 4 and 5 may, may not
or may only be partially combined since the interpretation of the results made by the same investigator who conducted the investigation
would have to be taken into consideration by the group or the individual
charged with formulating decisions. Steps 4 and 5 may be considered
as representing a phase denoted as the toxicological evaluation which
will fall into the direct task entrusted to expert groups.

In the light of findings in the documents reviewed, it appears logical to visualize the assessment of toxicity of food additives as a complex process having a dynamic rather than a static character, since
new scientific findings may at any time challenge the results of pre-

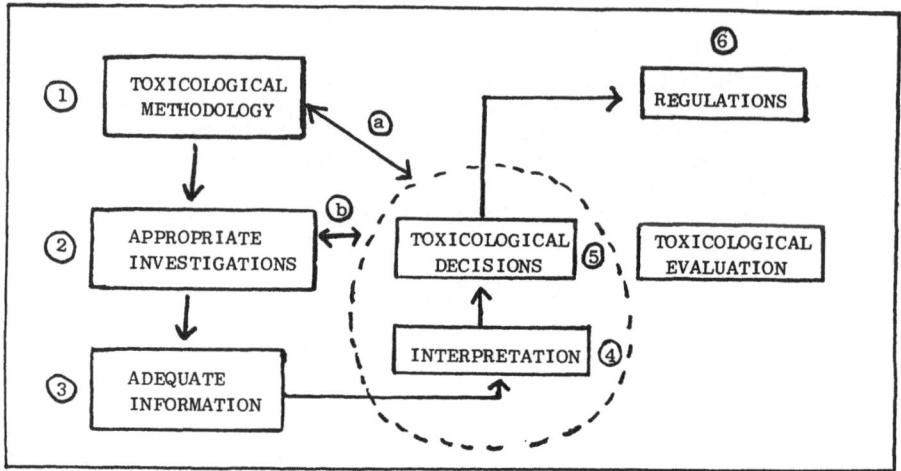

<u>Fig 1.</u> Flow diagram identifying the critical points and objectives of toxicological assessment of intentional and unintentional food additives.

vious evaluations. The two-way arrows a and b in the diagram, are intended to point this aspect.

It should be observed however, that the diagram in Fig 1 holds true only under the definition of the objectives indicated, i. e. regulations on the safe use. In reality, the intent of safety evaluations has been much wider in scope. Among other methods of evaluation, the assessment of consumer hazards has also been approached by encouraging the undertaking of estimations of potential food additive intake, total diet surveys and other studies aimed at assuring that the toxicological acceptable levels of intake are not exceeded by the average population. Furthermore, the toxicological decisions carried out by the WHO play an important role in the elaboration of international food standards carried out by the Codex Alimentarius Commission.

Over the years the process of safety evaluation of food additives has adopted certain approaches which can be summarized in the following sequence of decisions:

a. Acceptance of a no-effect level established in the course of some appropriately conducted long-term test or tests in laboratory animals;

b. Application of an arbitrary safety factor which, in the opinion of the experts, was in keeping with the nature of the compound being evaluated, given the circumstances of its intended use and with the quality of the experimental studies available;

c. Allocation of unconditional, conditional, or temporary acceptable daily intakes (ADIs), where appropriate, on the basis of considerations set forth.

6.2 The No-Effect Level(s)

From the various investigations a dosage level can be established that causes no demonstrable effect in the animal used (167). The essential basis of evaluation in almost every case is one or more long-term studies and most useful quantitative index is the highest dosage level that causes no significant effect either in acute, short-term or long-term studies. In some cases a particular dosage level is found to have only one effect, the significance of which from the toxicological point of view might be doubtful. Some effects, such as osmotic action at high dosage levels, may be properly disregarded in an evaluation of the toxicity of a lower dosage range. The decision to disregard a particular effect in a series of studies must be made by scientists experienced in this field. In general, it is advisable, when in doubt, to err on the side of regarding as significant an effect that may later be found to be unimportant, rather than to disregard an effect that may later be shown to be relevant. It has been a fairly common practice in the past to regard interference with weight gain as of no significance if a corresponding reduction in food intake was demonstrated on the grounds that the effect was due to interference with palatability. However, statistically significant interference with weight gain should not be lightly disregarded. The dosage level at which no significant toxicological effect was observed is expressed as mg/kg of body weight per day for a stated animal special (168, 169).

There is a need to consider more closely what "no-effect" means. The obvious intention is that the maximum dietary level that causes no deleterious effect should be taken for extrapolation to give the acceptable dietary intake in man. It may be difficult, however, to know whether an effect observed is deleterious or not. For example, diarrhea may be toxic effect, or it may be due to the osmotic effect often associated with a high dose level of the test substance. Decrease of weight gain may be due to toxic anorexia or to a loss of palatability of the diet. If effects of a physical nature (such as osmosis) or other effects (such as a palatability defect or stimulation of the metabolizing enzymes in the liver) resulting from a high dose level of the test substance, but unrelated to its toxic action, are included with toxic effects in selecting the "no-effect" level, it is reasonable to apply a lower margin of safety than that required for an unequivocal toxic effect.

In the absence of adequate evidence to the contrary, it should be assumed that any effect observed is a toxic effect. The onus for establishing that an effect observed is not a toxic one must rest on the investigator. Such features as reversibility and the differentiation of effects at lower dose levels may assist in distinguishing between physiological and pathological phenomena. Research aimed at elucidating problems of this nature should be encouraged (170).

When applied to data from animal experiments, the term "no-effect level" refers to the level of a substance that can be included in the diet of a group of animals without toxic effects. With certain substances, the highest level that can be incorporated in a diet fails to produce any effect. However, some food additives do exert toxic effects when fed at high levels and for these the maximum no-effect level is used. The maximum no-effect level should be determined in the most appropriate animal species and be based on the most pertinent criteria of toxicity.

A variety of effects, in the present state of knowledge, are not deemed to be of toxicological significance, provided they are fully attributable to normal physiological adjustment and are reversible. They include for example, changes in intestinal flora, laxative effects due to bulk or osmotic load, caecal enlargement and diminished growth rate caused by high levels of non-digestible substances, and liver hypertrophy and induction of microsomal enzymes due to gross overloading with certain metabolizable substances (171).

6.3 Margin of Safety, Safety Factors and the Problem of Extrapolating from Animal Data to Man

Undoubtedly, adequate evidence from human studies is the most satisfactory for the assessment of the human hazard. However, many difficulties arise in conducting such experiments and, for this reason, reliance must be placed on other forms of evidence. So far as the animal experiments are concerned, the use of high dosage levels of the test substance and the spread of the investigations over a number of different species make it reasonable to extrapolate the data applicable to man.

From these various investigations a dosage level can be established that causes no demonstrable effect in the animals used. In the extrapolation of this figure to man, some margin of safety is desirable to allow for any species difference in susceptibility, the numerical differences between the test animals and the human population exposed to the hazard, the greater variety of complicating disease processes in the human population, the difficulty of estimating the human intake and the possibility of synergistic action among food additives.

It is inescapable that some arbitrary factor must be applied in order to provide an adequate margin of safety. Where the maximum ineffective dose in animals is calculated in mg/kg body weight, a safety factor of the order of 100 has been widely used. In the absence of any evidence to the contrary, it is believed that this margin of safety is adequate.

The accuracy with which the maximum ineffective dose in animals can be defined clearly varies with the data that can be obtained. Where the proposed additive has a low toxicity, it may not be possible to demonstrate any adverse biological effect. Provided that any effects which might be predicted on the basis of current knowledge have been satisfactorily excluded, the hundredfold margin of safety may also be applied to the maximum ineffective dose administered in such cases. This clearly limits the possible daily level of use of a food additive. This margin of safety covers most of the substances so far proposed as additives. However, further consideration might have to be given in specific cases involving relatively inert substances (172).

Some margin of safety is necessary for the extrapolation of the maximum dietary level causing no effect in experimental animals to the acceptable dietary intake in man. An arbitrary factor of 100 has been widely accepted and this figure has been previously recommended (172). In practice the margin of safety has varied from 10-fold to 500-fold, based on the scope and comprehensiveness of the data available.

It is not necessary to demand the rigid application of an arbitrary figure. There are several grounds upon which variation of a safety margin might be applied. For example, in the case of an additive for which an adequate amount of toxicological data is not available or in situations where temporary acceptable daily intakes are recommended, a larger margin of safety should be employed.

Another example that may be cited is when the food additive is proposed for use in food items that show wide variations in daily intake, perhaps for climatic reasons, such as ice cream or soft drinks. Again, some foods may be particularly popular with children and this may be thought to justify an increase in the safety margin (173).

The magnitude of the margin of safety to be applied is technically a factor of the adequacy of available toxicological data. If an intentional food additive is a beneficial constituent of the diet or is a normal body constituent, this may provide grounds for a lower safety margin. It would not be feasible to apply a 100-times safety margin to many common food additives, e. g. , sodium chloride. There are also many substances, some of which may be used as food additives, that are known to be well tolerated by man at certain dose levels. Valid human data should take precedence over predictions arrived at the extrapolation from animals studies and may make it possible to apply a lower margin of safety.

When pertinent biological data (such as acute and long-term toxicity, biochemical reactions and histopathology) reveal a uniform species response, and when the most sensitive criterion of effect is clear-cut and the effect is reversible, then a materially reduced margin of safety can and should be applied to the "no-effect" level. Another example is the the situation where the "no-effect" level of a product is based on cholinesterase inhibition or adaptive liver enlargement. In these cases the margin of safety may be reduced substantially below the usual 100-fold margin of safety, provided that the additional biological data are satisfactory. In no case, however, should this factor be employed to justify the use of amounts of the additive in excess of that required for the indicated purpose.

The margin of safety to be applied to the "no toxic effect" level in the process of extrapolation from animal data to human exposure is fundamental for deriving values such as the acceptable daily intake.

It is important, therefore, that all details of the animal data and probable exposure be carefully evaluated. Continued research in this area is to be encouraged. Exploratory research in additional animal species, new techniques and new biological systems may yield data unique in character that are of research value but that should not necessarily be used to determine the "no toxic effect" level. Only when such data become recognized as significant should they be prime factors of evaluation.

It may be concluded that the 100-fold margin of safety is a useful general guide. It should not be applied rigidly and under certain conditions it may be increased or decreased. However, when a margin of safety other than the 100-fold margin is used, the basis for the change should conform to the principles outlined above (174).

More recently, it has been stated that in the extrapolation of animal data to man, the application of a safety factor is required for the following reasons: (a) to allow for any differences in sensitivity between the animal species and man; (b) to allow for wide variations in sensitivity among the human population; and (c) to allow for the fact that the number of animals tested is small compared with the size of the human population that may be exposed. A safety factor of 100 has been widely accepted. But it would be unreasonable to apply this figure too rigidly, for example, in the case of substances that are normal constituents of the human diet or are normal intermediary metabolites. When there are adequate data to show that a substance in the human body is converted by digestion or metabolism to a normal constituent of the diet, or that a substance is not absorbed from the gastrointestinal track, these data are used in the evaluation. When toxicological data derived from experiments in man are available, they may be used to provide a lower safety factor since they obviate the need for interspecies extrapolation.

On the other hand, there may be reasons to increase the safety factor--for example, when the amount and/or the quality of toxicological information are limited. Furthermore, the nature of the toxic effect produced by an additive at very high levels might demand an increase in the factor in order to ensure safety in use.

From the above exposition it may be construed that the figure of 100 represents a safety factor which when applied to the "no toxic effect" levels found in experimental animals it would increase 100-fold the margin of safety (or it will give a 100-fold safety margin) in the process of extrapolation from animal data to human exposure for the purposes of deriving values such as acceptable daily intakes (ADIs).

6.4 Acceptable Daily Intakes (ADIs) and Other Important Toxicological Decisions

The expression "acceptable daily intake" has become part of the terminology concerning the evaluation of food additives as well as the assessment of toxicity of pesticide chemicals. The above expression has often been condensed into an acronym (ADI) without connotation other than brevity and it has been extensively used to denote either a concept or a figure expressed in terms of milligram per kilogram body weight (mg/kg bw). The concept of acceptable daily intake is based on the widely accepted fact that all chemicals are toxic but their toxicities vary markedly, not only in nature, but also in the amount that is required to produce signs of toxicity. The figure (mg/kg bw) is derived from experimental data in laboratory animals and/or appropriate observations in man (176).

A detailed historic account of the evolution of the concept of the ADI and of how its present meaning became established over the years, while historically illustrative and intellectually challenging, may generate some degree of confusion to the non-initiated. Thus, in order to facilitate the historical research for the academically minded reader and at the same time to avoid misunderstandings for the more practically minded reader, after a brief historical outlook, the current definitions of ADI and other important toxicological decisions will be given in the form of a glossary.

6.4.1 Historical Outlook

At the very outset considerations were given to establish basis for evaluating the safety of use of food additives at a specified level of intake (177) or possible daily level of use of a food additive (178). These levels should be established on the maximum ineffective doses in animals. However, any attempt to establish a safe dose for carcinogenic substances in the human diet at present would be unwise (179). Acceptable levels should be proposed as acceptable intake zones which should be divided into unconditional and conditional daily intake zones for man (180). A zone of acceptability represents the limit of intake that can be regarded as presenting no significant hazard to health on the basis of the evidence available. The conditional zone of acceptability represents levels of use of food additives that can be employed safely, but at which it is thought desirable that some degree of expert supervision and advice should be readily available. The unconditional zone of acceptability represents levels of use that are effective technologically and can be safely employed without expert advice (181).

However, the use of two zones of acceptability, having regard to all the circumstances, in the case of food colors are neither desirable nor required (182). Overall zones of acceptability are divided into two parts: unconditional and conditional and at the same time acceptable daily intake has usually been expressed as milligram of the substance in question per kilogram of body weight.

There are, however, certain food additives that are more appropriately limited in terms of levels of treatment--for example, flour-treatment agents. There are also certain additives that are common components of food or normal body constituents. In such cases it is unreasonable to set specific limits. The appropriate method of expressing acceptable levels of use must be decided in each case (183).

The acceptable daily intake is the daily dose of a chemical that appears to be without appreciable risk on the basis of all the facts known at the time. "Without appreciable risk" is taken to mean the practical certainty that injury will not result even after a lifetime of exposure.

Many factors have to be considered in deriving from the dose level that causes no toxicological effect in an experimental animal an estimate of the acceptable intake in man. It is necessary to take into account species differences, individual variations, incompleteness of available data, and a number of other matters. It must be remembered that food additives may be consumed by people of all ages throughout the whole lifespan, that they are eaten by the sick as well as the healthy, and that there are wide variations in individual dietary patterns. Each case must be judged on its own merits.

It will be observed from the above that the acceptable daily intake is only an estimate and depends upon a great number of factors, all of which should be taken into consideration. Therefore an exact maximum acceptable daily intake cannot be calculated. This is one of the reasons why, in some cases, the zone of acceptability is divided into two parts--"conditional" and "unconditional." Although the whole zone of acceptability may be safely used, obviously the smaller the amount of a given chemical consumed, the smaller the risk. However, there are circumstances where one has to weigh one risk against another. For a food color, for instance, one would be inclined to make the acceptable risk smaller than for an antimicrobial used to preserve food that is scarce in many parts of the world. The conditional zone is one that can be safely used under certain conditions, which are specified where appropriate. Thus, in some cases, the use of the chemical might also be permitted for a limited length of time in order to obtain information from further work. In cases where the conditions are not specified, a final decision on whether intakes that fall within the range of conditional acceptance may be considered acceptable in particular circumstances should be taken by a group of scientists, including a toxicologist experienced in this field (184).

However, the conditional zone of acceptability is not to be confused with the conditional (temporary) ADI which is established on toxicological information not fully adequate by current standards and to which a safety margin greater than usual is applied (185).

Toxicologically, it generally makes no difference how a chemical is distributed in the diet provided that the overall content does not exceed the acceptable daily intake (ADI). If the levels proposed are likely to result in overall amounts in the diet equal to the ADI, difficulties might arise from the presence of this chemical in other foods. A problem of this sort might arise from background levels, spray drift or other causes. It is advisable to reserve some small proportion of the ADI to cover this situation (186).

If the toxicological information for the evaluation of safety is not adequate, it is suggested that some substances, especially those that are urgently needed or are present in relatively minute amounts, might be given at least temporary clearance. Thus, the establishment of "temporary acceptable daily intakes" is recommended in situations in which a particular food additive would be useful, or may already be in use, and for which toxicological or other data are not fully adequate to permit an acceptable daily intake to be set by the normal procedure. The conditions that need to be satisfied before such a "temporary acceptable daily intake" is established are as follows:

a. Each chemical additive must be considered on its merits;
b. The temporary ADI must be established only for a specific and definite period, namely, 3-5 years;
c. In setting a temporary ADI, the additional biochemical and toxicological data required for the eventual establishment of an ADI must be clearly stated. The additional requirements must be justified as being essential for the protection of the consumer;
d. A review of the original and new data must be carried out before the expiration of the provisional period (187).

In the evaluation of flavoring substances and non-nutritive sweetening agents the following terms were used: <u>unconditional ADI</u>, <u>conditional ADI</u> and <u>temporary ADI</u>.

An <u>unconditional ADI</u> was allocated only to those substances for which the biological data available included either the results of adequate short-term and long-term toxicological investigations or information on the biochemistry and metabolic fate of the compound or both.

A <u>conditional ADI</u> was allocated in either of the following two circumstances:

a. When the data fell short of the requirements for an unconditional ADI and specified further work that was required;
b. For specific purposes arising from special dietary requirements.

A <u>temporary ADI</u> was allocated when not quite enough data were available to fully establish the safety of the substance and it was considered necessary that the additional evidence be provided within a stated period of time. If the further data requested do not become available within the stated period, it is possible that the temporary ADI will be withdrawn in the future.

The fact that an ADI for an additive was not established (either because adequate data were lacking or the available information was unsuitable) should not be interpreted as casting doubt on the safety of the substance nor should it be considered tantamount to a recommendation for its withdrawal from use (188). Acceptable daily intakes (ADIs) were established when adequate information was available. It was further decided to use the terms "unconditional ADI," "conditional ADI," and "temporary ADI," where appropriate, in the evaluation of the antibiotics.

An unconditional ADI was allocated only to those substances for which the biological data available included the results of adequate short-term and long-term toxicological investigation and information on the biochemistry and metabolic fate of the compounds. A conditional ADI was allocated either for specified uses or when the data fell short of the requirements for an unconditional ADI. A temporary ADI was allocated if the available data, while indicating that the use of a given substance is likely to be safe, were considered inadequate to justify a final conclusion. In such cases, the additional evidence required should be submitted within the stated time limit, or the conditional acceptance of the substance may be withdrawn (189).

The previous practice in allocating ADIs was followed. That is an unconditional ADI was allocated only to those substances for which the biological data available included either the results of adequate short-term and long-term toxicological investigations or information on the biochemistry and metabolic fate of the compound, or both.

A conditional ADI was allocated for specific purposes arising from special dietary requirements.

A temporary ADI was allocated when the available data were not fully adequate to establish the safety of the substance and it was considered necessary that the additional evidence be provided within a stated period of time. If the additional data requested do not become

available within the stated period, the temporary ADI may be withdrawn by a future session of the committee.

Whereas all ADIs are subject to periodic review, especially when
additional data are available, reconsideration of temporary ADIs is
obligatory after the date specified. The decision arrived at will depend
on the information available at the time of review. It is not intended
to maintain indefinitely the temporary status of ADI for a food additive.

For those additives for which the available information was grossly
inadequate to establish safety, no ADI was allocated. It was further
observed that these decisions are naturally subject to revision in the
light of new evidence (180).

Certain food additives have a very low toxicity and their level of
use in foods is limited if good manufacturing practice is followed,
consequently these additives do not require the establishment of a
definite ADIs (191, 192).

On the other hand, it is inappropriate to attempt to set ADIs for
heavy metals and to trace contaminants. In these cases a different approach is needed and provisional tolerable weekly intakes were established for the heavy metals such as mercury, lead and cadmium
(193, 194).

Several modifications on previous decisions were subsequently done
and a new definition to the ADI given. In effect, the acceptable daily
intake (ADI) for man, expressed on a body-weight basis, is the amount
of food additive that can be taken daily in the diet, even over a lifetime,
without risk. (It was recognized that the expression 'ADI' in terms of
body weight does not reflect the relative exposure of animals of different size as accurately as would the metabolic mass, which is equal
to $W_b^{0.75}$, but it was also recognized that in practice, the method of
expressing the dose in terms of mg/kg body weight has proven satisfactory.)

An ADI is allocated only to substances for which the available data
include either the results of adequate short-term and long-term toxicological investigations or satisfactory information on the biochemistry and metabolic fate of the compound, or both.

An ADI may be allocated temporarily, pending the provision of
additional data within a stated period of time. This measure implies
that the toxicological data are adequate to ensure the safety in use of
the additive during the time for which the temporary ADI applies. If
the additional data requested do not become available within the stated
period, the temporary ADI may be withdrawn at a future meeting of
the committee.

An ADI without an explicit indication of the upper limit of intake
("not limited") may be assigned to substances of very low toxicity,
especially those that are food constituents or that may be considered
as foods or normal metabolites in man. An additive having a "not
limited" ADI must meet the criteria of good manufacturing practice--
for example, it should have proven technological efficacy and be used
at the minimum level of efficacy, it should not conceal inferior food
quality or adulteration, and it should not create a nutritional imbalance.

There may be circumstances in which the ADI is not applicable.
Thus it may be exceeded for special dietary purposes--for example,

in the case of modified celluloses, to reduce the energy content of the diet. On the other hand, the ADI for glutamic acid and glutamates does not extend to foods for infants under three months old.

Previously, a conditional ADI was allocated to a number of substances, often in addition to an unconditional ADI. Variations in the rules for applying conditional ADIs have given rise to some confusion. For this reason, it was considered that the allocation of conditional ADIs should be abandoned.

ADIs are intended as guides only and may be exceeded, after consultation with experts, in circumstances in which there may be important advantages in doing so. An ADI provides a sufficiently large safety margin to ensure that there need be no undue concern about occasionally exceeding it provided the average intake over longer periods of time does not exceed it (195). Other toxicological conclusions relate to postponing a decision, no allocation of ADI and declare that a substance should not be used (196).

Finally, the expression "ADI not limited" should be discontinued and instead the expression "ADI not specified" should be used. This expression should, each time, be accompanied with the following explanatory note:

"This statement means that, on the basis of available data (chemical, biochemical and toxicological), the total daily intake of the substance arising from its use or uses at levels necessary to achieve the desired effect and from its acceptable background in food, does not, in the opinion of the committee, represent a hazard to health. For this reason, and for reasons stated in the individual evaluations, the establishment of an acceptable daily intake (ADI) expressed in mg per kg of body weight is not deemed necessary" (198).

Conclusions regarding the evaluation of the carcinogenic risk are summarized (3) in the following way:

The term "carcinogen" has caused confusion because it applies to agents that are so varied in their quantitative and qualitative characteristics that their control requires many different approaches. However, common usage would seem to necessitate retention of the term. Chemical carcinogens can vary in potency in comparable test systems by a factor as high as 10 (7).

Since all chemical carcinogens pose a hazard, human exposure must be reduced to the feasible minimum. With compounds such as aflatoxin that may be active in microgram doses, the achievement of this objective may raise formidable practical difficulties.

The action of the majority of carcinogenic compounds is associated with preliminary changes (e. g., hyperplasias, cirrhosis) the role of which is not clear. However, there are some chemicals that give rise to neoplasms only after the induction of particular pathological effects. For example, the cancers of the urinary bladder observed in rats treated with Myrj 45 (polyoxyethylene monostearate) are thought to have been caused by the presence of bladder calculi induced by the chemical rather than by its direct action. A no-effect level for chemicals that produce tumors in this way may be established.

The evaluation of the carcinogenic effects of administered hormones must take into account their endogenous occurrence and participation in the regulation of physiological functions. If an intake of a hormone does not increase its level beyond the physiological range, then it probably represents a no-effect level. The endocrine status of the test species used should be as close as possible to that of man.

The induction of cancer by some carcinogens is attributable to their physical characteristics. For example, some forms of asbestos are carcinogenic in man and animals. This appears to be related to the physical characteristics of the fibers.

In summary, therefore, it would seem logical that tumor induction be considered as a manifestation of toxicity to be studied as an individual problem in each instance. In some cases, the data available may permit the logical determination of a tolerance level, whereas in others, currently the great majority, no such approach is possible.

From a practical standpoint, there is sometimes an irreducible environmental background level of certain cancer inducing compounds, such as aflatoxins and polycylic aromatic hydrocarbons. The toxicologist must take this into account in his evaluation and recommendations (198).

Consequently, in those situations where carcinogens are unavoidable, or where the banning of a substance would impose a hardship or an unrealistic economic burden, the toxicologist must assess the risks associated with different levels of exposure. Proposed approaches for such evaluation include those made by Mantel & Bryan (199) and by Albert & Altshuler (200). All the proposals suffer from lack of sufficient data to establish their validity and/or from arbitrary assumptions that lead to unrealistic estimates. Friedman has proposed the incorporation of the equivalent of a reference standard to make relative assessments possible. This whole area is of great practical importance and it is suggested that WHO should convene a separate meeting to evaluate this subject (201).

6.4.2 Current Important Toxicological Decisions

Below are listed and summarized the most important conclusions and decisions regarding the toxicological aspects of food additives which are presently used in assessing safety.

ADI for man: The acceptable daily intake (ADI) for man, expressed on a body weight basis, (mg/kg bw) is the amount of a food additive that can be taken daily in the diet, even over a life time, without risk. It is allocated only to substances for which the available data include either the results of adequate short-term and long-term toxicological investigations or satisfactory information on the biochemistry and metabolic fate of the compound, or both (202).

Temporary ADI: An ADI may be allocated temporarily, pending the provision of additional data within a stated period of time. This measure implies that the toxicological data are adequate to ensure the safety in use of the additive during the time for which the temporary ADI applies. If the additional data requested do not become available within the stated period, the temporary ADI may be withdrawn at a future meeting of the committee (202).

ADI not specified: An ADI without an explicit indication of the upper limit of intake may be assigned to substances of very low toxicity, especially those that are food constituents or that may be considered as foods or normal metabolites in man. This expression was adopted as a more suitable expression than "ADI not limited" which was previously used. An additive having an "ADI not specified" must meet the criteria of good manufacturing practices--for example, it should have proved technological efficacy and be used at the minimum level of technological efficacy, it should not conceal inferior food quality or adulteration, and it should not create a nutritional imbalance. The above expression means that, on the basis of available data (chemical, biochemical and toxicological), the total daily intake of the substance arising from its use or uses at levels necessary to achieve the desired effect and from its acceptable background in food, does not represent a hazard to health. For this reason, and for reasons stated in the individual evaluations, the establishment of an acceptable daily intake expressed in mg/kg body weight is not deemed necessary (203).

Conditional ADI: In previous deliberations of the committee "conditional ADIs" were allocated to a number of substances, often in addition to "unconditional ADIs." Variations in the rules for applying conditional ADIs have given rise to some confusion. For this reason, it was considered that allocation of conditional ADIs should be abandoned (204). However, certain food additives (146) awaiting reevaluation maintain both conditional and unconditional ADIs.

No ADI allocated: This expression is applicable to substances for which the available information is not sufficient to establish their safety or when the specifications for identity and purity are not adequate (205). The fact that an ADI for an additive was not established should not be interpreted as casting doubt on its safety nor should it be considered for its withdrawal for use (206).

Not to be used: This expression is applicable to substances for which there is sufficient information on which to base such decision (205).

Decision postponed: This expression is applicable to cases when to precise information is available concerning matters related to technology use (205).

Acceptable level of treatment: Acceptable daily intakes are usually expressed as milligrams of the substance in question per kilogram at body weight. There are however, certain food additives that are more appropriately limited in terms of levels of treatment (207). See, for example, flour treatment agents (207).

Acceptable residues: Acceptable residues in human food have been established for antibiotics found in foods (208).

Provisional tolerable weekly intake: This decision was established because it was found inappropriate to attempt to set ADIs for heavy metals such as mercury, lead and cadmium. In retrospect, it is plain that the concept of an ADI for any substance is based on the assumption that each day's intake is ultimately cleared from the body and that, for the most part, such clearance is rapid and complete (unless the com- gives rise to biotransformation products that enter into intermediate metabolism). Exceptions to this general rule have been encountered and have involved the storage of low levels of lipophilic compounds in the body fat of man. Further more, ADIs are intended to be used in allocating the acceptable amounts of an additive to specific intended uses where it will serve necessary technological purposes and will be employed in accordance with good manufacturing practice. Such concepts are inapplicable to trace contaminants.

In view of the above considerations, a new approach is needed in dealing with heavy metal contamination of food. Therefore it has been allocated a provisional tolerable weekly intake for each of the metal contaminants considered. The basis for this approach was as follows:

a. The contaminants are able to accumulate within the body at a rate and to an extent determined by the level of intake and by the chemical form of the heavy metal present in food. Consequently, the basis on which intake is expressed should be more than the amount corresponding to a single day. Moreover, individual foods may contain above-average levels of a heavy metal contaminant, so that consumption of such foods on any particular day greatly enhances that day's intake. Accordingly the provisional tolerable intake is expressed on a weekly basis.

b. The term "tolerable," signifying permissibility rather than acceptability, is used in those cases where intake of a contaminant is unavoidably associated with the consumption of otherwise wholesome and nutritious foods, or with inhalation in air.

c. The use of the term "provisional" expresses the tentative nature of the evaluation, in view of the paucity of reliable data on the consequences of human exposure at levels approaching those with which the committee is concerned.

ADIs are intended as guides only and may be exceeded, after consultation with experts, in circumstances in which there may be important advantages in doing so. In the opinion of the committee, an ADI provides a sufficiently large safety margin to ensure that there need be no undue concern about occasionally exceeding it provided the average intake over longer periods of time does not exceed it. In addition there may be circumstances in which the ADI is not applicable (210).

This list of decisions has been compiled by utilizing the most recent documents. If it appears to the reader rather extensive and complex, this is also so because, over the years, the committee has extended its scope to include the evaluation not only of intentional food additives but also of certain antibiotics, trace elements, food contaminants and processing aids. Consequently, there have been some minor changes in its approach to the problem of toxicological evaluation, especially with respect to the allocation of acceptable daily intakes.

6.4.3 Exclusion from the ADI of Amount Occurring Naturally in Foods

The rule that the ADI should not include amounts of a substance naturally present in food has been followed since the sixth meeting of the committee and was restated in the seventeenth report (204).

In principle, however, the toxicity of a substance is the same whether it is naturally present in the food or added subsequently. Moreover, it is not normally possible to differentiate by chemical analysis between a substance naturally present and added quantities of the same substance. It was therefore agreed that, as a general rule, the ADI should include the total amount of a compound in food. However, there are exceptions, and each case should be considered individually. As a corollary, the need was stressed to verify the total amount of the substance under study in the diet of experimental animals. If, however, the substance occurs in food in a chemical form different from that employed as a food additive the two quantities may have to be evaluated separately (211). Ascorbic acid, benzoic acid and nitrates were examined in the light of this new position. In addition, formic acid, sorbic acid, tocopherols, free glutamic acid, and their salts are other examples of food additives whose present ADIs are not considered to cover the amounts naturally present in food (212).

6.4.4 Applicability of ADIs to Children

In dealing with the problem of exposure of infants and children to contaminants in food, it was pointed out that one reason why it was inappropriate to set ADIs for the heavy metals, lead, cadmium and mercury was that the special susceptibility of the fetus, the newborn child and the young child could not be accurately expressed. It was also pointed out that children can be considered a high-risk group in relation to lead exposure and consequently the provisional tolerable weekly intake of 3 mg of lead per person did not apply to infants and children. The special problems relating to the exposure of infants and children to contaminants in food should be studied in depth by appropriate expert bodies.

Scientific evidence, much of it derived from animal experiments and supported by clinical observations, indicates that newborn and very young children are particularly sensitive to the harmful effects of foreign chemicals. Among the reasons for this are the immaturity of enzymatic detoxifying mechanisms, incomplete function of excretory organs, low levels of plasma proteins capable of binding toxic chemicals, and incomplete development of physiological barriers such as the blood-brain barrier. Moreover there appears to be a general vulnerability of rapidly growing tissues, which is particularly important with regard to the developing central nervous system.

Concerning the question of whether or not the ADIs allocated to food additives can be applied to all age classes including newborn, infants and young children, it was felt that the safety factors used for the determination of ADIs provide for individual variations in metabolism and sensitivity to foreign chemicals. Thus, for most food additives, the ADIs are applicable to all children older than 12 weeks. In this respect, toxicological and metabolic studies of food additives should always include investigations that permit the evaluation of safety for the newborn and the infant (239).

6.4.5 Administrative Overtones

It has been observed that the assessment of the toxicity of a food additive should be thought of as having a dynamic character. This is particularly true with regard to the assessment of the toxicity of those food additives which, because of their nature and use, need to be kept under constant review. In addition, new information may become available and may require a revision of the toxicological decision previously made. In the current terminology this situation is referred to as "re-evaluation of a substance." This task has frequently required the adoption of administrative attitudes designed to ensure the continuous awareness of parties interested in generating scientific data and aimed at establishing the safety of food additives. The adoption of temporary ADIs, the indication of further work required and/or desirable and the establishment of deadlines for submission of this work, are a few examples of such administrative measures.

It is of interest to note the remarks done with regard to the further work requested on a particular food additive. It has been agreed to request only work that is urgently needed in the interests of safety. All other suggestions for further work that may seem desirable, but not so urgently needed, have been so indicated. Attention of manufacturers and users of food additives was drawn to the fact that, in the future, if a statement is issued about further work being required, this matter should given urgent attention. If the additive in question is one that is already in use, its continued use will be supported only if the further work required has been carried out and the results justify continuance of the use of the additive. If no action is taken to provide the further evidence that is required, it will be assumed that neither the manufacturers nor the users are interested in continuing the use of the additive. In this case, it may well be decided to recommend the prohibition of its use. If the food additive is a new substance not yet in use and if further work has been required, a conditional intake level may be established for a limited period to allow the results of this additional work to be submitted and studied (213, 214).

6.4.6. Estimation of Food Additive Intake

It will be useful to try to define the standard daily dietary dose. This is taken to be the amount of the food additive that might be expected to be consumed by an average adult eating a normal diet as determined from some appropriate dietary survey. It should be assumed in these calculations that all the foods likely to be treated with the additive will contain it at the level proposed (215).

It is desirable that national governments should maintain a check on the total intake of each food additive, based on national dietary surveys, to determine whether the total load in the diet approaches the acceptable daily intake. Toxicologically, it generally makes no difference how a chemical is distributed in the diet provided that the overall content does not exceed the acceptable daily intake (ADI). In some instances, regulatory bodies may decide to recommend the use of a particular chemical in certain specified foods. If the levels proposed are likely to result in overall amounts in the diet in excess of the ADI, difficulties might arise from the presence of this chemical in other foods (216).

6.5 The Concept of Irreducible Levels for Contaminants in Food

The increasing sensitivities of the analytical methods developed in recent years have led to the detection of large numbers of hitherto unsuspected compounds in foods in minute amounts. In this respect it was emphasized that the presence per se of a trace amount of a toxic substance in food does not indicate hazard to man. The health hazard to man can only be determined by taking into account both toxicological knowledge and information about potential exposure. However, in the case of potent carcinogens, for example certain mycotoxins, it was recommended that efforts should be made to limit their presence in food to irreducible levels. An irreducible level was defined as that concentration of a substance which cannot be eliminated from a food without involving the discarding of that food altogether, thus severely compromising the ultimate availability of major food supplies (236).

6.6 Impact of New Scientific Methods on Safety Evaluations

In previous reports, reference was made to the rapid progress in the biological and chemical sciences, and it was stressed the need for toxicologists to use this knowledge for a better assessment of safety of chemical substances. In recent years many new toxicological approaches have been developed. Rapid developments are in progress for example in the areas of in vitro and in vivo assessment of mutagenic and carcinogenic effects. In addition to pharmacology, the use of electron microscopy, histochemistry, cytochemistry, immunopathology, biochemistry, molecular biology, and behavioral sciences are being used for the evaluation of toxicological processes in many laboratories.

These scientific approaches are of great importance since they often provide more insight into mechanisms and thus allow a more realistic extrapolation to man, particularly when utilized in conjunction with detailed information on absorption, distribution, metabolism and excretion of the compounds under study.

It should be pointed out that many biological methods are very sensitive, and permit recognition of clearly discernible effects at levels that are orders of magnitude below those causing changes demonstrable in conventional toxicological studies. Consequently, the "no-effect levels" obtained in such studies will often be much lower than those found in conventional studies.

In many toxicological tests, compounds are applied by routes that do not correspond to ingestion in the diet by man. Moreover, the results of some tests are qualitative rather than quantitative, and this makes it difficult to correlate them with other experimental data.

In evaluating data from unconventional tests it is particularly important to use flexibility and scientific judgement and not to be rigid in applying safety factors and assigning ADIs (236).

6.7 The Need for International Laison in Safety Evaluations

The fact was noted that there are several international groups involved in the toxicological evaluation of food additives, and that the conclusions of these groups sometimes differed from those of the Joint FAO/WHO Expert Committees on Food Additives. Such discrepancies could be due to different interpretations of the data, but generally they arise because of a difference in the data available for safety evaluation. It was therefore recommended that if an international group has new substantial data and consequently arrives at an evaluation of a compound different from that of the above mentioned international committee, then these data should be requested and the compound should be re-evaluated promptly by the Joint FAO/WHO Expert Committee on Food Additives. However, mechanisms to effect a better laison between various expert groups in order to assure a greater degree of uniformity of the various evaluations should be sought (236).

7. SOURCES AND NATURE OF INFORMATION

The importance of publishing experimental results has been continuously emphasized. Progress in work on food additives would be helped if more relevant experimental results were published in scientific journals. In many instances these results remain available only to a restricted group. If the cooperation of those sponsoring these investigations could be assured, the international organizations might consider the possibility of preparing lists of unpublished reports with a view to making them more widely available, on request, to workers in this field (217).

Work that is published in the scientific literature is subject to scientific examination, criticism, refutation or confirmation. Unpublished reports, on the other hand, are not necessarily submitted to this scrutiny. For this reason, when considering scientific literature, much greater weight will usually be given to published than to unpublished work. It is an accepted principle that published information is preferred as the basis for toxicological decisions and preference will always be given to published work (218).

There is an urgent need for more complete publication of the experimental work carried out in this field and also for an improvement in the facilities necessary to achieve this (219, 220).

The need was reaffirmed for adequate relevant information for preparation of specifications and toxicological evaluation. It was therefore recommended that Member Governments requesting an evaluation of a food additive, either directly or through the Codex Alimentarius Commission, should supply the necessary information including the technological function for which the substance is used (221).

The need has also been stressed for a more effective laison with the chemical and food industries in order to obtain information as complete as possible on methods of manufacture and of specifications for the substances under consideration and on their uses. It is recommended that the International Union of Pure and Applied Chemistry should be asked to assist in facilitating this exchange of information (222).

8. SOME EFFECTS OF FOOD ADDITIVES

8.1 Hypersensitivity reactions

A number of food additives are known to cause allergic manifestations in susceptible individuals. Sometimes these are due to occupational exposure and the evidence obtained in such instances is used in assessing allergenicity. No approval should be given for the use as a food additive of a substance causing serious or widespread hypersensitivity reactions. For food additives with an allergenic potential, the inclusion on food labels of lists of the individual additives used has been suggested as a means of enabling sensitive individuals and their physicians to identify the possible sources of allergic reactions. The practicability and effectiveness of such a measure is uncertain and the matter requires further consideration (223).

Some evidence of possible hypersensitivity reaction has been observed in the case of menthol (224) and the risk of allergic reactions connected with some enzyme preparations used both in human medicine and food technology has been pointed out (225).

8.2 Persorption Phenomena

The possibility exists that particular additives that have hitherto been regarded as totally unabsorbed, since they are, for practical purposes, completely insoluble, may be taken up by a process of persorption. Although excretory mechanisms are known to exist for some persorbed materials, clarification of this aspect is necessary.

Information on the tissue uptake and storage of macromolecular materials is frequently lacking. In the case of propylene glycol alginate, labelled with ^{14}C either in the alginate or propylene glycol moiety, whole-body autoradiography of treated mice served to establish lack of absorption of the alginate. Unlike lipid-soluble substances whose storage within the body is nonspecific, some macromolecular materials are localized within lysosomes of cells of the reticuloendothelial system. Degraded carrageenan behaves in this way and is retained in the sites of storage, for example in Kupffer cells of rhesus monkeys, for six months or longer after administration has ceased. The consequences of uptake and storage of macromolecular substances in reticuloendothelial cells are not well understood, but there is some indication that alterations of phagocytic function may occur.

In view of the availability of a range of techniques (analytical histochemical, ultrastructural, and autoradiographic) to supplement light-microscopic observations, further studies to obtain information on the tissue storage of macromolecular food additives should be carried out (226).

8.3 Carcinogenic Risk

Information on a number of food additives and food contaminants considered as part of the scientific background which deals with the available evidence on the potential carcinogenic risk can be found (227).

Many points of interest were revealed from the examination of food additives and contaminants being suspected of carcinogenic effects. The most important are:

a. The apparent lack of information on the toxicity or potential carcinogenicity of many food additives;
b. The inadequacy of the design, execution and interpretation of some experiments or of reported information in some of the publications in this field and the frequent lack of corroborative evidence;
c. The need for detailed pathological evaluation of any lesion observed in experimental studies;
d. The difficulties arising in interpretation of local sarcoma formation at the site of injection;
e. The difficulty of completely excluding at the present time carcinogenic contaminants from food, from processes used in the preparation of food, and from substances coming into contact with food;
f. The possibility that some natural constituents of the diet or even an essential nutrient, such as selenium, may constitute a carcinogenic risk. Clearly these substances cannot be completely excluded from the diet;
g. The difficulty of carrying out and interpreting epidemiological studies;
h. The wide variety of food colors, many of which do not appear to have been adequately tested included in the permitted lists of different countries;
i. The necessity of separate assessment of the carcinogenic risk for each individual substance (228).

The potential carcinogenic risk has been discussed together with the mutagenic risk in (3) in relation with environmental chemicals.

8.3.1 The Mechanism of Mutagenesis

It is now accepted that the genetic material of all living organisms, with the exception of some viruses, is DNA. The genetic information is encoded in the sequence of base-pairs such that three bases specify one protein amino acid. The code is said to be universal, meaning that the same three bases (triplets) correspond to the same amino acid in all living systems. The double helical structured DNA proposed by Watson and Crick has made it possible to explain replication of the genetic material and mutations in chemical terms (229).

A number of chemicals, including alkylating agents, analogues of DNA bases, and other types of molecule have been shown to induce mutations in biological systems, ranging from viruses to mammals.

More recently the possible hazard to man from the presence of mutagenic chemicals in the environment has been recognized.

Mutations are classified as gene or point mutations, which may result from changes in one or a few bases, and as microscopically visible changes in the structure or number of chromosomes, which involve changes in many more bases. Point mutations may arise either by base substitution or frame-shift mechanisms. Base substitution can occur by incorporation of base analogues into the DNA, leading to mispairing on subsequent replication or by chemical reaction with a base already present in the DNA chain, giving rise to an abnormal base, which mispairs at the next replication. Frame-shift mutation involves addition or deletion of bases in the DNA and is induced by agents that, because of their size and shape, can become intercalated between the base pairs.

Heritable visible chromosome aberrations may follow exposure of cells to chemical mutagens. There are cellular mechanisms that can repair lesions in DNA. The importance of DNA repair processes in human disease is illustrated by the rare condition xeroderma pigmentosum, which is genetically determined and in which cellular repair of DNA lesions induced by ultraviolet light is defective (230). Sufferers from this disease have a greatly increased incidence of active skin tumors (231).

8.3.2 The Mechanism of Carcinogenesis

Many, perhaps most, chemical carcinogens are thought not to be carcinogenic themselves but to require metabolic activation in the body to form active products which induce cancer. This activation is usually mediated by tissue enzymes, which occur mainly, but not exclusively, in the liver. Sometimes, however, activation is mediated by enzymes of the microbial flora of the intestinal tract. The terms precarcinogen, proximate carcinogen and ultimate carcinogen have been introduced by Miller & Miller (232) to describe respectively, the compound administered, its metabolites with increased carcinogenic potency, and the final metabolic product that is thought to react with a cellular component or components to induce the malignant transformation. In spite of the very varied chemical structures of the known precarcinogens there is evidence that many of them are converted in the body to electrophilic reactants which interact with various nucleophilic centres in the cell, including nucleic acids, proteins, and protein-bound methionine. Similar conclusions apply to the metabolic activation of some mutagenic chemicals.

The need for metabolic activation of some carcinogens and mutagens has important implications for the design of in vitro tests for both activities. With some chemicals positive results can only be obtained in the presence of suitable metabolic activating systems.

Although the facts of interaction of the active forms of chemical carcinogens with cellular macromolecules are well established, the significance of these interactions for carcinogenesis is not yet understood. Reaction with DNA gives support for the idea that cancer can result from mutation of a somatic cell and thus for a close interrelation between carcinogenesis and mutagenesis. This is no more than a hypothesis, however, and various epigenetic mechanisms of cancer resulting from interaction with cellular RNA or proteins have been put forward. Recently, there has been much renewed interest in the idea that chemical carcinogens may activate latent tumor viruses already present in the cell. The above considerations probably apply only to those carcinogens that react covalently with cellular macromolecules (233).

REFERENCES

1. WHO/FAO Procedures for the testing of intentional food additives to establish their safety for use. Second Report. FAO Nutrition Meetings Report Series, No. 17; Wld Hlth Org. techn. Rep. Ser., No. 144, 1958.
2. WHO Procedures for investigating intentional and unintentional food additives. Report of a WHO Scientific Group. Wld Hlth Org. techn. Rep. Ser., No. 348, 1967.
3. WHO Assessment of the carcinogenicity and mutagenicity of chemicals. Report of a WHO Scientific Group. Wld Hlth Org. techn. Rep. Ser., No. 546, 1974.
4. Ref. 1, p. 13.
5. WHO/FAO Evaluation of the toxicity of a number of antimicrobials and antioxidants. Sixth Report. FAO Nutrition Meetings Report Series No. 31; Wld Hlth Org. techn. Rep. Ser., No. 228, p. 4, 1962.
6. WHO/FAO Specifications for the identity and purity of food additives and their toxicological evaluation: some emulsifiers and stabilizers and certain other substances. Tenth Report. FAO Nutrition Meetings Report Series, No. 43; Wld Hlth Org. techn. Rep. Ser., No. 373, pp. 28-30, 1967.
7. WHO/FAO General principles governing the use of food additives. First Report. FAO Nutrition Meetings Report Series No. 15; Wld Hlth Org. techn. Rep. Ser., No. 129, pp. 4-5, 1957.
8. WHO/FAO Evaluation of Certain Food Additives: Some Food Colors, Thickening Agents, Smoke Condensates and Certain other substances. Nineteenth Report. FAO Nutrition Meetings Report Series No. 55; Wld Hlth techn. Rep. Ser., No. 576, p. 6, 1975.
9. WHO/FAO Toxicological evaluation of certain food additives with a review of general principles and of specifications. Seventeenth Report. FAO Nutrition Meetings Report Series, No. 53; Wld Hlth Org. techn. Rep. Ser., No. 539, p. 6, 1974.
10. Ref. 7, pp. 5-6.
11. Ref. 7, pp. 7-8.
12. Ref. 5, p. 13.
13. Ref. 9, p. 6.
14. Ref. 7, pp. 8 and 11.
15. Ref. 9, p. 7.
16. WHO/FAO Evaluation of Certain Food Additives. Twentieth Report. FAO Food and Nutrition Series No. 1; Wld Hlth Org. techn. Rep. Ser. No. 599, pp. 8-9, 1976.

17. Ref. 7, p. 12.
18. Ref. 7, p. 14.
19. Ref. 16, p. 9.
20. WHO/FAO Evaluation of food additives. Some enzymes, modified starches and certain other substances: toxicological evaluations and specifications and a review of the technological efficacy of some antioxidants. Fifteenth Report. FAO Nutrition Meetings Report Series, No. 50; Wld Hlth Org. techn. Rep. Ser. , No. 488, pp. 30-31, 1972.
21. Ref. 7, p. 10.
22. WHO/FAO Specifications for identity and purity of food additives (Antimicrobial preservatives and antioxidants). Third Report. These specifications were subsequently revised and published as Specifications for identity and purity of food additives Vol. I. Anitmicrobial preservatives and antioxidants, Rome. Food and Agriculture Organization of the United Nations, pp. 3-6, 1962.
23. WHO/FAO Specifications for the identity and purity of food additives and their toxicological evaluation. Food colors and some antimicrobials and antioxidants. Eighth Report. FAO Nutrition Meetings Report Series, No. 38; Wld Hlth Org. techn. Rep. Ser. , No. 309, pp. 6-8, 1965.
24. Ref. 7, p. 10.
25. Ref. 22, p. 3.
26. Ref. 23, p. 6.
27. Ref. 23, pp. 6-7.
28. Ref. 6, p. 31.
29. Ref. 22, pp. 3-4.
30. Ref. 23, p. 7.
31. Ref. 6, p. 32.
32. Ref. 22, p. 4.
33. Ref. 22, pp. 4-5.
34. Ref. 23, pp. 7-8.
35. Ref. 6, pp. 31-32.
36. Ref. 22, p. 5.
37. WHO/FAO Specifications for the identity and purity of food additives and their toxicological evaluation: some antimicrobials, antioxidants, emulsifiers, stabilizers, flour-treatment agents, acids and bases. Ninth Report. FAO Nutrition Meetings Report Series, No. 40; Wld Hlth Org. techn. Rep. Ser. , No. 339, p. 10, 1966.
38. Ref. 6, p. 13.
39. Ref. 9, p. 11.
40. Ref. 5, p. 5.
41. Ref. 37, p. 10.
42. Ref. 6, p. 13.
43. WHO/FWO Specifications for the identity and purity of food additives and their toxicological evaluation. Emulsifiers, stabilizers, bleaching and maturing agents. Seventh Report. FAO Nutrition Meetings Report Series, No. 35; Wld Hlth Org. techn. Rep. Ser. , No. 281, p. 18, 1964.
44. Ref. 2, p. 8.

45. Vettorazzi, G. and P. Miles-Vettorazzi. Safety evaluation of chemicals in food. Toxicological data profiles. I. Carbamate and organophosphorus pestidices used in public health and agriculture. Bull. Wld Hlth Org. , 52, Suppl. 1-61, 1975.
46. Ref. 7, pp. 9-10.
47. Ref. 23, pp. 8-9.
48. Ref. 8, pp. 10-11.
49. Ref. 36, p. 8.
50. Ref. 20, p. 7.
51. Ref. 43, p. 6.
52. WHO/FAO Specifications for the identity and purity of food additives and their toxicological evaluation: some food colors, emulsifiers, stabilizers, anti-caking agents, and certain other substances. Thirteenth Report. FAO Nutrition Meetings Report Series No. 46; Wld Hlth Org. techn. Rep. Ser. , No. 445, p. 26, 1970.
53. WHO/FAO Evaluation of food Additives. Specifications for the identity and purity of food additives and their toxicological evaluation: some extraction solvents and certain other substances: and a review of the technological efficacy of some antimicrobial agents. Fourteenth Report. FAO Nutrition Meetings Report Series, No. 48; Wld Hlth Org. techn. Rep. Ser. , No. 462, p. 6, 1971.
54. Ref. 8, p. 9.
55. Ref. 9, p. 7 and 25.
56. Ref. 8, pp. 7-9.
57. Ref. 2, pp. 4-5.
58. Ref. 1, p. 5.
59. Ref. 9, p. 30.
60. Ref. 1, p. 6.
61. Ref. 9, p. 9.
62. Ref. 1, p. 8.
63. Ref. 2, p. 8.
64. WHO/FAO Evaluation of the carcinogenic hazards of food additives. Fifth Report. FAO Nutrition Meetings Report Series. No. 29, Wld Hlth Org. techn. Rep. Ser. , No. 220, p. 8, 1961.
65. Ref. 1, pp. 8-9.
66. Boyland, E. The determination of carcinogenic activity. Acta Un. Int. Cancr, 13, 271, 1957.
67. Ref. 64, pp. 8-9.
68. USA National Research Council, Food Protection Committee. National Academy of Sciences Public, 749, 1959.
69. Ref. 64, pp. 10-12.
70. Ref. 1, p. 10.
71. Druckrey, H. Principles of toxicological methods, Arztl-Forsch. , 7, 449, 1957.
72. Ref. 64, pp. 12-13.
73. Ref. 64, pp. 13-14.
74. Ref. 64, p. 12.
75. Ref. 1, pp. 15-16.
76. Ref. 2, pp. 12-14.
77. Ref. 2, p. 23.
78. Ref. 1, p. 5.

79. Ref. 2, p. 7.
80. Dixon, R. L., Shultice, R. W. & Fouts, J. R. Factors affecting drug metabolism by liver microsomes. IV. Starvation. Proc. Soc. exp. Biol. (N. Y.), 103, 333, 1960.
81. Kato, R. & Gillette, J. R. Effect of starvation on NADPH-dependent enzymes in liver microsomes of male and female rats. J. Pharmacol. exp. Ther., 150, 279, 1965.
82. Friedman, L. Nutritional status and biological response. Fed. Proc., 25, 137, 1966.
83. Hotzel, D. Dtsch. Med. Forsch., 2, 105, 1964.
84. Tannenbaum, A. Nutrition and cancer. In: The Physiopathology of cancer, Homburger, F. Ed., 2nd ed., New York, Hoeber-Harper, p. 517, 1959.
85. Ref. 2, pp. 12-13.
86. Ref. 64, pp. 17-18.
87. Ref. 2, p. 13.
88. Ref. 2, p. 23.
89. Ref. 2, pp. 11-12.
90. Ref. 20, pp. 33-34.
91. Ref. 20, p. 34.
92. Ref. 2, p. 12.
93. Ref. 1, pp. 7-8.
94. Ref. 2, p. 8.
95. Ref. 64, pp. 7-8.
96. Ref. 9, p. 31.
97. Ref. 6, p. 35.
98. Ref. 5, p. 8.
99. Ref. 1, p. 13.
100. Ref. 9, p. 31.
101. Ref. 1, p. 14.
102. Ref. 37, p. 9.
103. Ref. 6, p. 12
104. Ref. 9, p. 32.
105. Ref. 2, pp. 14-15.
106. Ref. 2, pp. 23-24.
107. Ref. 1, p. 9.
108. Ref. 9, p. 30.
109. Ref. 5, p. 7.
110. Ref. 6, p. 35.
111. Ref. 1, pp. 10-11.
112. Ref. 1, pp. 11-12.
113. Ref. 5, p. 8.
114. Ref. 6, pp. 35-36.
115. Ref. 2, pp. 13-14.
116. Ref. 9, p. 33.
117. Ref. 2, p. 17.
118. WHO Principles for the testing of drugs for teratogenicity. Report of a WHO Scientific Group. Wld Hlth Org. techn. Rep. Ser., No. 348, 1967.
119. Ref. 2, pp. 16-17 and 24.

120. WHO Evaluation and testing of drugs for mutagenicity: principles and problems. Report of a WHO Scientific Group. Wld Hlth Org. techn. Rep. Ser. , No. 482, 1971.
121. Ref. 3, p. 9.
122. Ref. 3, p. 12.
123. Ref. 1, pp. 16-17.
124. Ref. 1, p. 5.
125. Ref. 64, p. 7.
126. Ref. 1, pp. 11-12.
127. Ref. 3, p. 8.
128. Ref. 3, pp. 8-9.
129. Ref. 9, p. 34.
130. WHO Principles for the testing and evaluation of drugs for carcinogenicity. Report of a WHO Scientific Group (Geneva 1968). Wld Hlth Org. techn. Rep. Ser. , 425, 1969.
131. Ref. 2, p. 9.
132. Ref. 2, p. 10.
133. Ref. 20, p. 34.
134. Ref. 5, p. 8.
135. Ref. 2, p. 9.
136. WHO Principles for pre-clinical testing of drug safety. Report of a WHO Scientific Group. Geneva 1966. Wld Hlth Org. techn. Rep. Ser. , No. 341, 1966.
137. Ref. 53, pp. 8-9.
138. WHO/FAO Pesticide Residues in Food. Report of the 1973 Joint FAO/WHO Meeting. Wld Hlth Org. techn. Rep. Ser. , No. 545, p. 9, 1974.
139. WHO/FAO Pesticide Residues in Food. Report of the 1974 Joint FAO/WHO Meeting. Wld Hlth Org. techn. Rep. Ser. , No. 574, pp. 8-9, 1975.
140. Ref. 16, p. 10.
141. Ref. 1, p. 5.
142. Ref. 1, pp. 14-15.
143. Ref. 5, p. 7.
144. Ref. 6, p. 35.
145. Ref. 9, pp. 30-31.
146. WHO/FAO Specifications for the identity and purity of food additives and their toxicological evaluation: some flavouring substances and nonnutritive sweetening agents. Eleventh Report. FAO Nutrition Meetings Report Series, No. 44; Wld Hlth Org. techn. Rep. Ser. , No. 383, p. 9, 1968.
147. Ref. 1, p. 15.
148. Ref. 2, pp. 17 and 24.
149. Ref. 2, pp. 18-19.
150. Stein, W. H. , Serrone, D. M. & Coulston, F. Safety evaluation of methoxychlor in human volunteers. Toxicol. appl. Pharmacol., 7, 499, 1965.
151. Sharrat, M. , Frazer, A. C. & Cutler, M. Methodological studies in the assessment of the acceptability of a food additive. In: Proceedings of the First International Congress of Food Science and Technology, New York, Gordon and Breach, p. 583, 1964.

152. Golberg, L. Liver enlargement produced by drugs: its significance. Proc. Europ. Soc. Study Drug Toxic. , 7, 171, 1966.
153. Ref. 2, pp. 15-16.
154. Ref. 2, pp. 17-18.
155. Ref. 53, p. 8.
156. Ref. 3, p. 12.
157. Ref. 64, p. 14.
158. Ref. 64, p. 15.
159. Ref. 64, p. 33.
160. Ref. 64, pp. 15-16.
161. Ref. 64, pp. 16-17.
162. Ref. 2, p. 19.
163. Ref. 64, p. 5.
164. Ref. 3, p. 12.
165. Ref. 3, pp. 9-11.
166. Vettorazzi, G. The safety Evaluation of Food Additives: The dynamics of toxicological decisions. Lebansm.-Wis, U.-Technol. , 8, 195, 1975.
167. Ref. 1, p. 17.
168. Ref. 5, pp. 9-10.
169. Ref. 6, p. 36.
170. Ref. 2, p. 20.
171. Ref. 9, p. 9.
172. Ref. 1, pp. 17-18.
173. Ref. 2, pp. 19-21.
174. Ref. 2, pp. 21-22 and 24.
175. Ref. 9, pp. 9-10.
176. Vettorazzi, G. State of the art of the toxicological evaluation carried out by the Joint FAO/WHO Expert Committee on Pestidice Residues. I. Organohalogenated pesticides used in public health a and agriculture. Res. Rev. 56, 197, 1975.
177. Ref. 7, p. 14.
178. Ref. 1, p. 18.
179. Ref. 64, p. 22.
180. Ref. 5, pp. 6 and 10-12.
181. Ref. 43, pp. 10-11.
182. Ref. 23, pp. 13-14.
183. Ref. 37, p. 9.
184. Ref. 6, pp. 36-37.
185. Ref. 6, p. 47.
186. Ref. 2, pp. 6-7.
187. Ref. 2, pp. 7 and 22.
188. Ref. 146. pp. 10-11.
189. WHO/FAO Specifications for the identity and purity of food additives and their toxicological evaluation: some antibiotics. Twelfth Report. FAO Nutrition Meetings Report Series, No. 45; Wld Hlth Org. techn. Rep. Ser., No. 430, pp. 14-15, 1969.
190. Ref. 52, pp. 8-9.
191. Ref. 52, p. 9.
192. Ref. 20, p. 8.

193. WHO/FAO Evaluation of certain food additives and the contaminants mercury, lead and cadmium. Sixteenth Report. FAO Nutrition Meetings Report Series, No. 51; Wld Hlth Org. techn. Rep.
Ser., No. 505, pp. 9-11, 1972.
194. WHO/FAO Evaluation of mercury, lead, cadmium and the food
additives amaranth, diethylpyrocarbonate and octyl gallate. FAO
Nutrition Meetings Report Series, No. 51A; WHO Food Additives
Series, No. 4, 1972.
195. Ref. 9, pp. 10-11.
196. Ref. 9, p. 12.
197. WHO/FAO Toxicological evaluation of certain food additives with
a review of specifications. Eighteenth Report. FAO Nutrition
Meetings Report Series, No. 54; Wld Hlth Org. techn. Rep. Ser.,
No. 557, p. 10, 1974.
198. Ref. 3, pp. 11-12.
199. Mantel, N. & Bryan, W. R. "Safety" testing of carcinogenic agents.
J. nat. Cancer Inst., 27, 455, 1961.
200. Albert R. E. & Altshuler, B. Considerations relating to the formulation of limits for unavoidable population exposures to environmental carcinogens. In: Proccedings of the Twelfth Hanford Biology Symposium on Radionuclide Carcinogenesis, Richland, Wash-
ington. C. L. Sanders, 1972.
201. Ref. 3, p. 12 and Annex.
202. Ref. 9, p. 10.
203. Ref. 9, pp. 10-11.
204. Ref. 9, p. 11.
205. Ref. 9, p. 12.
206. Ref. 146, p. 11.
207. Ref. 37, p. 9.
208. Ref. 189, p. 15.
209. Ref. 193, pp. 9-10.
210. Ref. 9, p. 10.
211. Ref. 198, pp. 8-9.
212. Ref. 197, pp. 10.
213. Ref. 37, p. 10.
214. Ref. 6, pp. 7 and 37.
215. Ref. 1, p. 17.
216. Ref. 2, p. 6.
217. Ref. 1, p. 7.
218. Ref. 37, p. 7.
219. Ref. 5, p. 7.
220. Ref. 197, p. 8.
221. Ref. 16, pp. 9-10.
222. Ref. 6, p. 9.
223. Ref. 197, p. 10.
224. Ref. 156, p. 6.
225. Ref. 20, pp. 10-11.
226. Ref. 52, p. 23.
227. Ref. 64, pp. 24-31.
228. Ref. 64, pp. 5-6.

229. Watson, J.D. Molecular biology of the gene, 2nd end. , New York, Benjamin, 662, 1970.
230. Cleaver, J.E. Defective repair replication of DNA in Xeroderma Pigmentosum. Nature, (Lond.) 218, 652, 1968.
231. Ref. 3, pp. 6-7.
232. Miller, E.C. & Miller, J.A. The mutagenicity of chemical carcinogens: correlations, problems and interpretations. In: Hollaender, A. ed. , Chemical mutagens, New York, Plenum, Vol. 1, pp. 83-119, 1971.
233. Ref. 3, pp. 6-8.
234. WHO/FAO Evaluation of certain food additives. Twenty-first report. FAO Food and Nutrition Series, No. 8; Wld Hlth Org. techn. Rep. Ser. , No. 617, pp. 10-11, 1978.
235. Cramer, G.M. , Ford, R.A. & Hall, R.L. Estimation of toxic hazard-decision tree approach. Fd Cosmet. Toxicol. (In publication), 1978.
236. WHO/FAO Evaluation of certain food additives. Twenty-second report of the Joint FAO/WHO Expert Committee on Food Additives. Wld Hlth Org. techn. Rep. Ser. (in publication), 1978.
237. Ref. 2, p. 15.
238. WHO/IARC Transplacental carcinogenesis. International Agency for Research on Cancer, Lyon, France. Scientific Publication No. 4, 1973.
239. Ref. 234, p. 10.

Chapter 2

General Principles in the Toxicological Evaluation of Pesticide Residues in Food

1. INTRODUCTION

At a meeting of a WHO Expert Committee on Pesticide Residues held jointly with the FAO Panel of Experts on the Use of Pesticides in Agriculture in 1961 (1) recommendation was made that studies be undertaken to evaluate possible hazards to man arising from the occurrence of residues of pesticides in foods. Following this meeting, which was endorsed by an intergovernmental meeting in Rome in 1962, Joint Meetings of the WHO Expert Committee on Pesticide Residues and the FAO Committee on Pesticides in Agriculture were held in 1963 (2) and 1965 (3). These meetings were concerned with establishing acceptable daily intakes for man (ADIs). The reports from these meetings and the supporting documents were then considered by the FAO Working Party on Pesticide Residues with a view to recommending maximum residue limits (tolerances) and appropriate methods of analysis.

Joint Meetings of the WHO Expert Committee on Pesticide Residues and the FAO/WHO Working Party of Experts on Pesticide Residues (also referred to as FAO/WHO Joint Meetings on Pesticide Residues or simply the Joint Meeting) have subsequently been held annually commencing in 1966. Accounts of these meetings, which are held alternatively in Geneva, Switzerland, and Rome, Italy, are contained in reports that have been published after each meeting. These reports outline the general principles and summarize conclusions reached and recommendations made in carrying out the evaluations of pesticide chemicals. They are supplemented by accompanying volumes which contain monographs with evaluations, comments, acceptable daily intake figures, and recommended maximum residue limits in food items, together with summaries of toxicological studies and chemical data for the individual pesticides considered at the meeting. The reports are published both by WHO and FAO separately (WHO Technical Report Series and FAO Agricultural Studies). Similarly the monographs are published by WHO and FAO separately (WHO Pesticide Residue Series and various FAO documents).

93

Pesticides are indispensable to the farmer in his fight against pests and diseases. Without their use, many foods could not be produced economically or perhaps at all, and the yield of all crops could be seriously reduced.

Pesticides vary widely in the degree of possible hazard they present to users, consumers of treated crops, farm animals, wildlife and the consumer. Obviously the concern is only with the possible hazards to human and animal consumers. However, aspects concerning the safety of the operator have already received, and continue to receive, the attention of WHO and ILO (International Labor Office) and of nature conservationists concerned internationally with the problem of protecting wild life against the effects of pesticides

A wide range of pesticide chemicals is needed for the control of pests and diseases on many types of food throughout the world. Frequently, the use of a pesticide for a specific purpose does not lead to a residue. In recording the belief in the basic principle that, as far as possible, food should be pure, it is recognized that, because of the necessity of using pesticides, residues may occur. It is, therefore, considered what measures should be taken to ensure that, if a residue is present, it will not harm the consumer. In particular it is noted the question of the applications of pesticides to stored food following harvest and emphasized the importance of using, if possible, compounds that leave either no residue or unquestionably harmless residues.

In those areas where pests have developed resistance to pesticides, high dosage rates have to be used to obtain adequate control.

It is also recognized that some pesticides such as sulfur present no real problem because, in world-wide experience over many years, they have shown themselves to be without serious hazard to man. No residue problem is presented by the use of pesticides on ornamental plants and nursery stock, or no crops which are not used for human or animal consumption at any stage (4). In discussing the legislative control of pesticide residues, the difficulties related to this problem are recognized and it is noted that a number of countries had already taken measures, of a varied nature, towards their solution.

In spite of the different national registration and control systems, some common patterns can be identified. Firstly, there is informal consultation between manufacturers and research and government departments concerned. Secondly, guidance, preferably of a detailed nature, is given to farmers on how to use pesticides so that any residues ultimately present in the food do not offer a hazard to consumers. Thirdly, punitive means exist to deal, if necessary, with farmers who, in ignorance or defiance of that advice, so misuse a pesticide that unnecessarily high residues remain in the food.

This common pattern can be put into effect in a number of ways as described in the four methods mentioned below, and it is for each country to decide the method most suitable to its own conditions and resources. Four requirements are basic to them all. They are: a. qualified official agricultural advisers who know the agricultural practice of the country, the chief crops and the pests and diseases of those crops, and who have an adequate working knowledge of the different types of available pesticides; b. analytical facilities for determining any residues on a crop grown, treated and harvested in that country; c. toxicological advice on the amount of a pesticide that may be consumed daily in the human diet without effect on the consumer; and d. finally, and most important of all, joint consultation by all authorities, agricultural, health, analytical and nature conservation, at all times to agree on the conditions for the use of a pesticide before that use is implemented. Knowledge of the national diet is also essential.

Whichever method is adopted, it is advisable for the authorities to obtain a preliminary evaluation of the effectiveness of a pesticide in their country before it is used commercially. Residue data should be obtained at the same time, and often the manufacturer who wishes to introduce the product may be in a position to make the necessary analyses.

Method 1. The importation and/or manufacture and use of selected pesticides are entirely controlled by government authorities. Firms are allowed to manufacture or import only certain pesticides. These are used only by the agricultural department on the advice of its qualified advisers. It is desirable that samples of treated foods be analyzed for residue content and that this analysis be continued until the authorities are satisfied that they have adequate knowledge of the residue level occurring in the food.

Method 2. The importation and/or manufacture of selected pesticides continues under government control. Their use on behalf of the government is extended to farmers who have been trained for this purpose and who will use them to the satisfaction of the advisory agricultural and health officials. Confirmation of correct use by residue analysis should be obtained if possible.

Method 3. Generally, there need be no hindrance to the importation and/or manufacture of pesticides, but all products offered for sale must be registered. The purpose of registration is to ensure, as far as possible, that the product will be effective and safe if used according to the directions on the label. The sale and use of pesticide products are limited to selected farmers. The selection will be made on the advice of competent authorities who must be satisfied that the farmer will use the pesticide as advised. This procedure will in effect have a restricting action on the range of pesticides manufactured or imported. Confirmation of correct use by residue analysis may be considered necessary in certain cases.

Method 4. All pesticide products are registered for sale, but the sale and use of the more toxic products are further controlled or even prohibited. With the exception of the requirement for registration, the sale and use of the less toxic pesticides are otherwise unrestricted. Official detailed advice on the correct use of pesticides is issued, and measures for dealing with those who misuse the products are available. Adequate analytical facilities must be available for residue determinations.

The official advice on the correct use of a pesticide should include information on one or more of the following: a. the edible crops to which its use is restricted; b. the maximum dose per application; c. the maximum number of applications; d. the last date of application (in the case of winter crops); and e. the minimum interval between last application and harvesting. The advice should appear on the label of the product and should be a condition of registration. All label claims and instructions for use should be as agreed by the competent authorities. Special attention should be paid to the labelling of seed grain treated with pesticides, such as the organomercurials and hexachlorobenzene, which are present at concentrations that will make the consumption of the grain harmful to man and farm animals. Official advice should also be disseminated through the advisory services and by means of advisory leaflets, trade journals and manufacturers' literature. The advice should also refer to operator precautions and the protection of farm animals, wildlife and the public.

To be effective, punitive measures against those who fail to observe the official advice should be on a mandatory basis. The measures may be based either on tolerances or on minimum intervals between last application and harvesting.

From the descriptions above, it is evident that, with limited funds available for the purpose, more satisfactory results would be achieved by spending these funds on an advisory service to the farmer on the use of pesticides, and on officials for checking that pesticides are being used correctly, than on extensive random sampling and analysis of food from the market. This course would permit the authorities to concentrate their available analytical facilities, devoted to enforcement, on foods which may be overtreated with pesticides as the result of unusual conditions (5).

2. CONSIDERATIONS ON THE PHYSICAL AND CHEMICAL IDENTIFICATION OF PESTICIDE CHEMICALS

Experimental studies are generally conducted on laboratory animals to assess any possible hazards arising from the consumption of pesticide residues. It is important that these experimental studies be performed upon material which is chemically identical with the toxic products which the pesticide will leave in human or animal food. To assure this, the chemical changes which the pesticide undergoes from exposure to air, moisture, the enzymes of crops and food, and animals, as well as any reaction between the pesticide and nutrients by which food may be altered, must be known. It is necessary that investigations be made, both with the pesticide and with its specific formulations under conditions of expected use. In the case of farm animals, it is of great importance to knownthe fate of a pesticide, and especially its rate of excretion in milk and its concentration in milk products, in eggs and in other animal products. This knowledge may lead to the prohibition of the use of a pesticide for treatment of farm animals or of their food and may require its replacement by a pesticide proved acceptable for this purpose (6).

Certain pesticides are of unknown or variable composition, e. g. , toxaphene and other chlorinated terpenes and technical grades of BHC. Consequently, it is often difficult to relate the existing toxicological data on these compounds to the products in actual agricultural use. This situation is likely to occur more frequently in the future as patent protection of various compounds expires, permitting them to be produced by a number of different manufacturers. If toxicological evaluations are to be applicable to products whatever their source, it is essential for such products to conform to specifications that ensure reasonable identity of composition. In this connection, attention is drawn to the WHO and FAO programs concerned with the development of specifications for pesticides and it is recommended that priority be given to specifications for pesticides that may result in residues in food. It is emphasized that for pesticides that are variable mixtures, it would be desirable, at some future date to have reference standards readily available from some central source (7).

Similar concern is expressed with regard to inadequate information on the composition of certain technical grade pesticides and associated contaminants, especially when the same chemical is produced by different manufacturers (8).

The question of the purity of technical grade of a number of pesticides is further discussed with relation to the possible influence of known and unknown impurities on the toxicity of the technical grades of the chemicals and of residues resulting from their use. Toxicological studies (both acute and chronic) are generally carried out with technical grade materials produced by commercial-scale process, and the resulting toxicological data normally take into account the presence of impurities. In view of the experience with 2, 3, 7, 8-tetrachlorodibenzo- b, e 1,4 dioxin and the finding several years ago of trace amounts in samples of 2, 4, 5-T, similar problems should be avoided. Admittedly, however, it is most unlikely that small amounts of unknown highly toxic impurities would be detected by chemical analysis of technical grade chemicals or formulations.

It was recognized that specifications such as those issued by FAO and WHO are seldom designed to take account of impurities occurring in technical grade pesticides at the trace level unless the importance of such impurities has already been revealed by biological studies. Such specifications are nevertheless valuable, and manufacturers should be encouraged to conform to them by producing the purest possible grades of pesticides consistent with constraints imposed by cost and scale of manufacture. Constant vigilance is, however, needed to detect reactions in workers at manufacturing plants, spray operators, animals, and plants that could give warning of possible toxic manifestations due to impurities.

Furthermore, it should be feasible and desirable to provide information on the setups used in industrial synthesis to aid in the forecasting the possibility that impurities of toxicological significance may be formed during manufacture. While difficulty of ensuring that this information is up to date and of drawing useful conclusions from it is recognized that an attempt should be made to include such information in future monographs (9).

Attention has recently been focused on the problem arising in connection with testing of technical products and the testing of formulations. Substances used in formulations may show toxic effects in their own right, alone or in association with the technical product. Their testing may provide additional supporting data on the toxicological aspects.

Specifically, if the basic toxicity of the active compound is altered
by the formulations or by changes in the purity of the technical product
in current use, further toxicological studies should be performed with
the new product (10).

The presence of nitrosamines has recently been reported in a number of pesticide formulations. Presently the problem is not completely
defined and its review has been deferred. However, sufficient information is available to indicate that the presence of nitrosamines can be
diminished if nitrite corrosion inhibitors are not added to the formulations. Additional information indicates that the nitrosamine content can
be minimized by modification of manufacturing processes, particularly
with respect to the sequence of nitration and amination steps (206).

3. CONSIDERATIONS ON TOXICOLOGICAL
TESTING PROCEDURES

No systematic elaboration on testing procedures was ever attempted
by the Joint FAO/WHO Meeting on Pesticide Residues. Instead it made
current use and took account of the principles and guidelines enumerated by various other expert groups as they appeared in the Second (11),
Fifth (12), Tenth (13), Eleventh (14), and Seventeenth (15) reports of
the Joint FAO/WHO Expert Committee on Food Additives, the report
of a WHO Scientific Group on Procedures for Investigating Intentional
and Unintentional Food Additives (16) and a WHO Scientific Group on the
Assessment of the Carcinogenicity and Mutagenicity of Chemicals (17).

In making reference to the programs of toxicological investigations
described, in, for example, the Second (18) and Fifth (19) reports of
the Joint FAO/WHO Expert Committee on Food Additives, the opinion
has been expressed that these programs should be considered as guides,
but the conduct of toxicological investigations remains the responsibility
of the competent expert. It is, however, believed that in the present
state of toxicological knowledge, such programs should be followed
when most new pesticides are being investigated, and it is hoped that
specific research and accumulated experience with the investigation of
pesticides will lead to new methods by which toxicological properties
can be discovered more surely and perhaps more expeditiously than
by following the mentioned programs (20).

In this respect, a recommendation has been issued that studies
should be promoted on methods used to assess the toxicity of pesticides
with the aim of improving the accuracy and speed of the assessment.
Examples of methods to be studied are those for determining percu-
taneous toxicity, and the effects of long-term exposure, including carcinogenicity (21).

During the course of its sessions, the Joint Meeting on Pesticide
Residues has occasionally commented on toxicological testing procedures and the main aspects touched upon are briefly described.

3.2 Aims of Toxicological Investigations

The aims of toxicological investigation are to ascertain: (1) the
amount of a pesticide to which man and farm animals can be exposed

daily for a lifetime without injury; (2) the nature of injuries which will
result if an excess is absorbed; (3) means for detecting subclinical
effects before they become injurious, (4) therapeutic measures for the
treatment of injuries; and (5) information which will allow workers to
utilize the pesticides safely.

These aims can be achieved only by the intelligent efforts of experienced qualified investigators who are not rigidly bound to follow a
schedule of required procedures. The procedures must be determined
by the chemical and physical properties of the pesticide, by its conditions of use and by its toxicological and biochemical actions, as they
are discovered during the progress of the investigation.

The aims enumerated above have been satisfactorily achieved for
pesticides now in use in those countries which exercise the most stringent control. This may not be the case for some pesticides in countries
with less stringent control, and whenever possible such investigations
should be undertaken or completed especially for new pesticides (22).

3.3 Animal Experiments

Before adequate observations upon man become available, experiments on animals would allow sound judgment towards the realization
of the primary aims (23).

3.4 New Methods for Toxicological Assessment

The development of new methods for toxicological assessment might
be taken into account in relation to pesticides already evaluated since
the toxicological decisions are necessarily conditioned by the methods
available at the time they are made. It should be recognized that the
development of a new method might, at any time, make it desirable
to review existing recommendations, whether or not they had been
made on a temporary basis. A need for re-evaluation may stem from
new information concerning residues or the identity of metabolites.
A re-evaluation may result in either raising or lowering the recommended safe limits.

The use of new methods may resolve anomalies and uncertainties
in data on particular pesticides and thereby provide greater assurance
concerning their safety, and may also provide information of value in
the toxicological evaluation of other pesticides and of other environmental chemicals (24).

3.5 Routes of Administration
(Gavage versus Feeding)

Results have been examined at short-term and reproduction studies
on several pesticides in which similar dosage levels of particular
compounds had been administered daily to groups of experimental animals by gavage and to other groups by incorporating the compound in
the diet. The need to expose experimental animals in a way that parallels human exposure has been discussed. Species such as the rat
normally feed more or less continuously during the night. When such

---

species are used for testing substances that act only briefly and that do not accumulate or produce cumulative effects, it is to be expected that dietary administration will cause less pronounced biological effects than administration by gavage, which permits the total daily intake to enter the body in a single dose. In almost every instance administration by gavage produces higher peak levels in blood and tissue than does incorporation in the diet.

In order to facilitate the interpretation of both feeding and gavage studies, attempts should be made to determine concentrations of pesticides and their metabolites in blood and tissue (25).

In examining further experimental data from studies where animals are fed a pesticide as part of the feed, it is again noted the obvious difference from data obtained in experiments where the compound is administered by gavage and the conclusion previously reached that experiments using gavage cannot replace feeding experiments for the testing of materials found or suspected of being found in food is reiterated (26).

3.6 Biochemical, Pharmacokinetic, and Metabolic Studies

Biochemical studies are important because they reveal the metabolism of the pesticide in the crop during the formation of the residue and subsequently in the animal which consumes it. It is important to know whether a substance is absorbed, its distribution in the body after absorption, its mechanism of action including its influence on enzyme systems, how it is metabolized, and the routes of final elimination. The toxicity of a pesticide may be altered at all these stages. In the crop or--in the case of veterinary pesticides--in the animal, a number of metabolites may be produced, some of which may be the active forms of the pesticide, as in the formation of paraoxon from parathion.

After ingestion, these active products may be further broken down to compounds that are excreted. Storage of these or of the parent chemical may occur. The fact that a compound appears to be rapidly broken down and excreted does not necessarily mean that it is more desirable as a residue than one which is stored, say, in the adipose tissue. Short-lived compounds formed during the breakdown might be very poisonous, whereas persistent compounds might be stored in an inactive form.

Broadly speaking, the more that is known of the fate and mechanism of action of a pesticide the better should be the understanding of its toxicity and consequently the easier it will be to set an acceptable daily intake for man (27).

Comparative metabolic studies may help in the development of new compounds. In effect, to be useful, pesticides must injure certain forms of life and it is generally presumed that they must be, in some degree, toxic to man. This is not necessarily true, as exemplified by the harmfulness of silica gel to certain insects. Workers on crop protection should strive to find new compounds with a selective toxicity towards a particular pest, while being essentially non-toxic to man (204).

Consequently, research should be encouraged into the differences between the normal metabolism of invertebrates, plants and warm-blooded animals as it relates to the susceptibility of these organisms to possible poisons. This information would be of value in the development of new compounds having a selective toxicity to a particular pest while being essentially non-toxic to man, farm animals and wild life (28).

In dealing with the use of biochemical parameters for establishing no-toxic effect levels, it is stressed the need for further discussion on the difficulties of distinguishing between significant toxic effects and adaptive responses. In particular, it is necessary to decide whether the changes associated with the induction of microsomal enzymes by a wide variety of exogenous compounds are to be regarded as a manifestation of toxicity. Previous induction of such enzymes may either increase or decrease the manifestation of toxicity attributable to exposure to a second exogenous or endogenous agent. There is a special need to consider this problem in relation to the possible effect of pesticides on the efficacy and toxicity of drugs given for medicinal purposes. These and related problems concerning chemical interaction between substances should be further investigated since only limited aspects of which were touched upon by a WHO Scientific Group (29) that met to discuss procedures for investigating intentional and unintentional food additives (30).

More recently, the role of pharmacokinetic studies in safety evaluation has been extensively explained. In effect it is now well appreciated that the tissue distribution, the mode and rate of metabolism, and the rate of excretion of a chemical may profoundly affect its toxicity. Furthermore, the rate of metabolic degradation of a pesticide in the environment influences its persistence. It has become the accepted practice in toxicological evaluation of pesticides to undertake studies of the biotransformation of the chemical and of its tissue distribution and excretion kinetics, generally after single dose administration.

Many pesticides and their metabolites, in addition to being excreted from the body in the urine, are also excreted in substantial amounts in the bile, as a consequence of which they may undergo enterohepatic recirculation. In addition, certain highly lipophilic substances may be distributed and stored in fat deposits after absorption from the gut. On repeated dosage these processes of absorption, metabolism, excretion and reabsorption become kinetically complex and may lead to the progressive tissue accumulation of a pesticide or one of its metabolites. This is especially likely where these chemicals are highly lipophilic, extensively biliary excreted and only slowly metabolized.

Studies of the pharmacokinetics of a pesticide during repeated low dosage are very desirable since they provide valuable information concerning possible accumulation or depletion and the probable maximum tissue concentration attainable. Such studies contribute to the safety evaluation of long-term exposure to pesticides at the low concentrations that are likely to be present in food (31).

3.7 Acute Toxicity Studies

The value of data on acute toxicity is that they give an idea of the inherent toxicity of the material (32).

3.8 Short-term Studies

Investigations covering less than half the animal's life span are included under this category. It is probable that the majority of toxic effects can be revealed in such studies (33).

3.9 Long-term Studies

These include tests covering the greater part of the animal's life span and research on the possible carcinogenicity of the residues.

These long-term studies are important for the determination of the dietary level of the compound which produces no effect, particularly when dealing with compounds that do not produce any measurable biochemical changes. Obviously such tests must be carried out on a species that has been shown by acute and/or short-term studies to be sensitive to the compound. If possible, the sensitivity should be similar to that of man and the metabolism of the compound in the animal should also be similar to that in man (34).

In stressing the need for analyzable number of animals it is observed that in the toxicological evaluation of several compounds, it proved difficult to interpret long-term studies because there were too few surviving animals at the end of the study for the results to be analyzed by appropriate statistical means. It is, therefore, suggested that experiments should be designed so as to permit valid statistical analysis (35).

The need for long-term studies for establishing no-effect levels has been emphasized on several occasions in implicit as well as explicit terms. Thus, in carrying out the toxicological evaluation of oxythioquinox (chinomethionat) it has been observed that because a no-effect level could not be demonstrated in long-term studies in the rat, no final assessment could be reached. Similarly, a safe limit has been established for endosulfan on the basis of adequate long-term studies and supporting data (36).

For the establishment of an acceptable daily intake for man, certain data, including data from long-term studies in at least one animal species, are normally required. The lack of such data usually precludes the establishment of an acceptable daily intake for man for a compound, even though long experience of its use suggests that it presents no hazard for man (37).

In the past, acceptable daily intakes for man have occasionally been established for pesticides for which the results of long-term studies in animals were not available. The general scientific literature contains an increasing number of examples of substances that have been presumed to be safe solely on the basis of chemical, metabolic, and short-term toxicological information, but that have subsequently been shown to exhibit toxic effects in long-term studies in laboratory animals.

It is therefore agreed that only in exceptional circumstances should an acceptable daily intake for man be established in the absence of satisfactory data from long-term studies in animals. For some organophosphorus pesticides it may still be logical to base an acceptable daily intake on data from adequate short-term in vivo studies of anticholinesterase activity, since such activity is the most sensitive criterion of effect for these compounds. Nevertheless, data from long-term experiments are usually required to provide assurance of the safety of moieties of molecules other than those responsible for the anticholinesterase activity (38).

These conclusions are stressed on subsequent occasions. A number of substances which were not found to be toxic in laboratory animals in short-term tests have subsequently shown toxic effects in long-term studies. Consequently, as a general rule, acceptable daily intakes for man should be established only when data showed that the possibility of a long-term toxic hazard had been substantially excluded. This will normally be the case only where data from long-term studies are available (39).

3.10 Special Studies (Carcinogenicity, Mutagenicity, Teratogenicity)

In evaluating the toxicological data on many pesticides, questions arise on the possible carcinogenicity, mutagenicity or teratogenicity of some of these compounds and on the interpretation of the relevance to man of some experimental animal results regarding these effects. Where a dose-response relationship in a teratogenicity test is found, it is felt that an evaluation can be carried out. Where problems of mutagenicity arise, it is agreed to accept the views stated in the report of the WHO Scienfitic Group on Procedures for Investigating Intentional and Unintentional Food Additives (16).

In discussing the question of possible carcinogenicity of some pesticides, no conclusive evidence for or against the carcinogenicity of those pesticides can often be achieved. Consequently, it is strongly urged that consideration be given to the question of dose-response for carcinogens and of possible threshold levels. A definite requirement in the assessment of carcinogenicity should be that experimental procedures follow the rules put forward in the Fifth Report of the Joint FAO/WHO Expert Committee on Food Additives (12) and the report on Carcinogenicity Testing published by the International Union against Cancer (40).

A recommendation is issued that WHO should convene a meeting of experts in the field of toxicology and carcinogenicity to consider the question of threshold levels and dose-response with respect to the carcinogenic potential of some pesticides and to evaluate the significance of carcinogenic effects of chemicals in experimental animals for assessing the potential risk of these chemicals to man (41).

The recommended meeting took place in subsequent years (17). More recently further recommendations in this field were issued. It is advised that evaluation of carcinogenic potential should be undertaken for those compounds which leave substantial residues on crops directly or indirectly used for human food. Evaluation of carcinogenic potential should also be undertaken on those pesticides which: a. have a chemical structure similar to known carcinogens, or closely related compounds; b. give rise to pathology which is suggestive of potential tumorigenicity; or, c. have pharmacokinetic properties suggestive or covalent binding to tissues or bioaccumulation (206).

The problem of nitrosatable pesticides is discussed and it has been observed that a number of N-nitroso compounds have been shown to exert a carcinogenic effect in animals. Recent experiments have demonstrated that N-nitroso compounds are formed from a number of nitrogen-containing pesticides in vivo as well as in vitro, and that in vivo formation may occur in man. Of the N-nitroso compounds formed from certain agricultural pesticides some are known to have a carcinogenic action in rodents. In recent studies such compounds have also been demonstrated to be mutagens in vitro.

The extent of formation of N-nitroso compounds in man, if indeed they are formed, is probably very limited, and it is not yet possible to predict the effect in man of low doses of these substances. It should be borne in mind that man is already exposed in the environment to a variety of other nitrosatable substances and carcinogenic nitrosamines. Further research should be conducted on the formation of N-nitroso compounds from pesticides under conditions and at concentrations that include those to which man might be exposed (42).

In further discussing the need for mutagenicity testing in the evaluation of a pesticide when estimating an acceptable daily intake for man, it is observed that the possible mutagenic action of chemicals has been already discussed by several WHO Scientific Groups (16, 17, 43). The importance of protecting the human population from exposure to mutagens in food is underlined. However, in view of the uncertainty about the extent to which most of the tests available at present are relevant for predicting the mutagenic hazard to man, no particular test to be required for estimating acceptable daily intakes for man can be recommended.

In spite of the difficulties in interpreting the significance for human health of the results from most tests for mutagenicity, it is agreed that such tests are desirable because they provide additional information on the biological activity of pesticides. Tests for mutagenicity are especially desirable in certain cases, e. g. , for substances that yield metabolites with stable carbonium ions or strong electrophilic reactivity.

Negative results from tests for other kinds of biological activity (e. g. , reproduction studies, teratogenicity studies, and carcinogenicity tests) give some assurance that the pesticide residue would not constitute a mutagenic hazard for man, especially when such negative results are obtained at dose levels very much higher than those to which man would be exposed.

The hope is expressed that research now in progress would lead to the development of mutagenicity tests known to be relevant to the predicting the mutagenicity hazard to man is undergoing rapid development and for this reason no particular test has been recommended. However, doses of the chemicals that bear some relationship to the concentrations likely to be encountered in food and the environment should be included in the range of doses used in mutagenicity tests.

Results of mutagenicity tests should be evaluated together with other toxicological data on each pesticide and more weight should be attached to the results of mutagenic tests in mammals than to those obtained from microbial or other non-mammalian systems or isolated cell systems. The significance of positive results from microbial tests, unsupported by information from tests of other kinds, would be regarded as uninterpretable for the purposes of establishing on acceptable daily intake for man. In addition, it was recommended that WHO should consider convening a special meeting to evaluate existing tests for mutagenicity with a view to predicting potential mutagenicity hazards to man and to recommend appropriate test procedures. In addition, this meeting should consider the possibility of establishing threshold intakes in relation to mutagenic action (47).

More recently, while awaiting for further information concerning the correlation between carcinogenicity and mutagenicity in vitro and in vivo, it has been stated that where a pesticide is shown to be a mutagen, carcinogenicity studies should be undertaken (206).

3.11 Special Studies (Dermal, Ocular, Inhalation Toxicity)

An investigation designed to evaluate the safety of food treated with a pesticide should also provide information concerning the protection of the health of workers. Studies should therefore include, for example, skin penetration of the pesticide (particularly as it may be influenced by formulation), skin irritation and sensitization, possible corneal injury, and, with some pesticides, injury following inhalation. The results obtained should provide the basis for the preparation of instructions on the safe handling in manufacture, formulation and application of that pesticide (48).

3.12 Observations in Man

Observations in man yield the soundest data for achieving the aims of toxicological evaluation. Every effort should be made to collect and to evaluate data on human exposure and on the presence or absence of human response during production, handling and agricultural study of a pesticide. Even after the pesticide has been introduced into commerce, observations on the exposure and response of workers are useful, particularly because workers are exposed to much greater amounts of pesticide than is the general population (49). Experience from workers exposed to pesticides could be valuable but has not so far been precise enough to assist in arriving at figures for acceptable daily intakes for man (50).

In reports of suspected cases of pesticide poisoning in man, details of the identity, the purity, the precise formulation, and the dose of the pesticides concerned and of possible concomitant exposure to similar or unrelated chemicals were often lacking. It is desirable to have further information about persons employed in the manufacture or formulation of pesticides, or in their application in the field. Such data would not only provide information of importance for the protection of personnel but, by indicating toxic effects specific to man, would be useful in assessing the safety of pesticide residues in food. The question of serious or fatal accidents due to exposure to certain pesticides could not be ignored and it is particularly necessary to discuss the actual and potential problems associated with exposure to such pesticides as diquat, paraquat and 2,4,5-T (51).

The hazard to man from the introduction of a chemical such as a pesticide into the environment can be more reliably predicted if information from carefully planned studies in man is available. Useful information may sometimes be derived from studies on persons who are occupationally exposed to the chemical or who have been accidentally poisoned by it. In these circumstances special efforts should be made to arrange for clinical investigations, including the analysis of samples of blood and tissue from the affected persons. Arrangements should also be made for the follow-up of exposed persons and for the collation of the data obtained. In some cases the exposed population may be large enough and sufficiently well defined to render appropriate epidemiological studies worthwhile. If effects that are apparently specific to man are observed, evidence obtained earlier from animal studies should be reassessed to see whether information has been overlooked or whether some different method of study might have been of greater predictive value.

Although there may be ethical and legal problems in carrying out investigations designed to establish safety or to detect toxicity in man, the use of volunteers may be justifiable when the administration of trace amounts can help in identifying metabolites. For instance, trials in man of those pesticides for which there is a known sensitive index of exposure (e. g. , cholinesterase inhibition) might be acceptable (52).

The evaluation of the potential hazards of pesticides and the allocation of acceptable daily intakes for man would be aided by knowledge of the human response to pesticide exposure. The various types of investigation and observation than can be made in man have been described in detail by a WHO Scientific Group (16). Such knowledge may in addition be helpful in revising protocols for animal studies to maximize their usefulness in predicting human response. To permit the development of data banks on human response to pesticide exposure, epidemiological studies should be designed that could yield data on both acute and chronic effects and accumulation in man. It was recommended that WHO seek the cooperation of the World Federation of Associations of Clinical Toxicology Centers and Poison Control Centers (Lyons, France) and others in developing such data banks (53).

It is highly desirable that the toxicological evaluation of pesticide residues in food be supplemented by information on occupational exposure and health effects. For this reason, such information should be published (54).

4. CONSIDERATIONS ON PRINCIPLES OF INTERPRETATION OF EXPERIMENTAL FINDINGS

Some specific problems encountered in the interpretation of experimental findings and on the significance of certain effects are discussed below.

4.1 Liver Tumors in Mice

The etiology and pathogenesis of liver tumors in mice has been discussed on several occasions (55-58).

Recent reports concerning a number of pesticides have highlighted the need for further information on the factors involved in the etiology and pathogenesis of liver tumors in mice. In many strains of mice, such tumors develop spontaneously, some with a relatively high incidence, in the absence of deliberate exposure to any test compound. Non-specific factors, such as calorie intake and dietary protein level and microbiological status profoundly affect the incidence of these tumors. Under these circumstances, it is difficult to be sure whether exogenous compounds that increase the risk of development of these tumors do so by facilitating events of natural origin and peculiar to the mouse as a species, or by inducing tumors that would not otherwise have arisen.

When tumors arise in the livers of dieldrin-treated mice, the cells of which they are composed show the same cytoplasmic change as surrounding non-tumorous liver parenchyma cells, namely, proliferation of the smooth endoplasmic reticulum. Apart from the latter manifestation, the liver tumors that arise in deildrin-treated and DDT-treated mice are similar to the liver tumors that arise spontaneously in untreated mice. Consequently, there is an urgent need for a better understanding of the nature, etiology, and pathogenesis of liver tumor development in mice (59).

WHO should consider investigating the significance of hepatoma development in mice for predicting the carcinogenic potential of certain pesticides for man, with special reference to dose-response relationships in hepatoma induction in mice and the possibility of threshold levels of exposure in tumorigenesis (60).

Consideration is given to the problem of interpreting data in respect of carcinogenicity where exposure of mice to a pesticide in food is associated with evidence of increased risk of development of liver tumors. Several organochlorine pesticides increase the risk of development of nodules in the livers of mice. It is not clear what proportion of the nodules are neoplastic but there is unequivocal evidence, in the case of some of the compounds, that they increase the incidence of neoplasms that metastasize to the lungs.

A feature of many substances (e. g. , phenobarbital) that increases the risk of liver tumor development in mice is that they induce microsomal drug-metabolizing enzymes and hypertrophy of the smooth endoplasmic reticulum of mouse liver cells. These biochemical and histological changes occur in the liver cells of other species but without associated tumor development. When tumors develop in the livers of mice that show these liver-cell changes, the biochemical and histological changes just referred to tend to be present in the tumor cells as well as in "normal" liver cells. Apart from this, the tumors that arise in response to exposure to chlorinated hydrocarbons are very similar in appearance and behavior to those that arise in untreated mice. It is known that in several strains of mice liver tumors, including some that metastasize to the lungs, may arise in untreated animals and that the rate may be as high as 100%. It was observed that there is a serious lack of knowledge regarding the processes involved in the development of liver tumors by mice and that it would be unwise to classify a substance as a carcinogen solely on the basis of evidence of an increased incidence of tumors of a kind that may occur spontaneously with such a high frequency.

In general, if the exposure of mice to a pesticide was associated with an increased risk of the development of liver tumors, long-term feeding studies on at least one other species should be required. Carcinogenicity tests in two species other than the mouse would be regarded as appropriate where it was evident that man might be exposed through food to a dose level close to one that increased the incidence of liver tumor in mice. Although the above considerations might be useful for general guidance, it would be essential for each pesticide to be considered and assessed individually (61).

More recently, in considering the re-evaluation of aldrin, dieldrin and chlordane, the formation of hepatomas by these compounds in certain strains of mice has been again considered. These liver tumors have not been found to develop in any species other than mouse as the result of exposure to dieldrin or chlordane and these chemicals have been shown to be nonmutagenic in a variety of studies. As previously observed, in many strains of mice liver tumors develop spontaneously at relatively high incidence and without intentional exposure to chemicals. These liver tumors arising in mice as the result of exposure to dieldrin or chlordane, or to other chemicals such as phenobarbital, are very similar in nature to the spontaneous tumors. The characteristic biological effects of chemicals which produce hepatomas in mice are the induction of the liver microsomal enzymes, proliferation of the endoplasmic reticulum and liver hypertrophy, all of which occur generally only at high dosage. These biochemical and cytological changes occur in other animals treated with these chemicals but liver tumors do not develop. In the rat the formation of liver tumors following exposure to a variety of chemicals would seem to correlate with degranulation of the endoplasmic reticulum of the liver cells and with subsequent changes in the microsomal enzymes (207). Degranulation of endoplasmic reticulum is known to be associated with carcinogenesis (208, 209, 212). Both dieldrin and phenobarbital degranulate the hepatic endoplasmic reticulum of CF_1 mice, a susceptible strain to dieldrin-induced tumorigenesis, but do not degranulate the endoplasmic reticulum of LAGG mice, a non-susceptible strain, nor that of rat or man.

A wide variety of halogenated organic compounds are known to produce this type of liver tumor in mice, which may be attributed in one or more of the following factors: a. the more rapid rate of metabolic

activation of these compounds in the mouse; b. potentiation of the tumorigenicity of the known high level of endogenous oncogenic viruses
in this species; c. genetic differences in the pathways of metabolism,
or d. genetic differences in the stability of the rough endoplasmic
reticulum. Metabolic dehalogenation of these compounds may give
rise to reactive intermediates which alter the enzymes of the endoplasmic reticulum, causing enzyme induction and membrane hypertrophy in most species, but possibly resulting in hepatic tumors in
mice. As previously stated, it would, consequently, be unwise to
classify a substance as a carcinogen solely on the basis of a species
strain-specific increased incidence of tumors of a kind that occur
spontaneously with high frequency. Where man might be exposed to a
chemical which resulted in an increased incidence of liver tumors in
mice, carcinogenicity tests in two species other than the mouse would
be appropriate. Such studies have been carried out for the compounds
mentioned above, in the rat and hamster, and these have shown no
evidence of increased tumorigenicity. Therefore, the production of
hepatic tumors by dieldrin and chlordane in the mouse is a species-
related phenomenon (206).

4.2 Stimulation of Microsomal Enzymes

During the past few years, evidence has become available that some
compounds stimulate the activity of microsomal enzymes in the liver
cells. These enzymes may affect the metabolism of other compounds.
The toxicological significance of the stimulation of the activity of liver
enzymes and of the associated morphological changes is difficult to
evaluate (62, 63).

WHO should examine the interpretation to be given to the effects of
pesticides on microsomal enzymes and should consider investigating
the significance of an interrelationship between liver enlargement,
stimulation of microsomal enzymes, and hepatoma, with respect to
predicting the health hazards of certain pesticides for man (64, 65).

4.3 Delayed Neurotoxicity Syndrome

A major toxicological problem long recognized to be associated with
such organophosphate esters as tri-o-cresylphosphate (TOCP) has been
brought to the attention in the evaluation of leptophos. This effect is
commonly known as "delayed neurotoxicity." This term refers to the
observations made on patients suffering from acute poisoning with
TOCP (and certain other organophosphorus compounds) of an apparent
recovery from the acute parasympathomimetic signs of poisoning followed by the onset after 8 to 14 days of clinical signs of ataxia, muscle
weakness and loss of appetite. Extensive reviews on the chemical
structure/activity relationship, biochemistry, and histological factors
relating to this syndrome have been published.

The delayed neurotoxicity syndrome affects only certain animal
species, including man. The most susceptible animal for laboratory
bioassay procedures, the adult hen, is not susceptible before 3 to 4
months of age. While the adult hen is the animal of choice for labora-

tory testing, cats, dogs, calves and sheep have also been shown to be susceptible. Some sub-human primates and rodents are resistant to both the clinical and the histological lesions. In contrast, man has been shown to be highly susceptible to the syndrome, as suggested by studies where occurrences of paralysis have been reported. Although no definite data are available, man may well be the most sensitive species exhibiting delayed neurotoxicity.

There are no known antidotes to delayed neurotoxicity, and recovery from ataxia is predominantly through development of collateral nerve pathways and physical therapy to develop muscles not served by affected nerves. Reference has been made in the literature to the induction of neurotoxicity by certain organophosphorus compounds used as pesticides and drugs. The dose in most experimental cases is high, and atropine, which protects against the short-term acute parasympathomimetic signs of poisoning, is ineffective against delayed neurotoxicity occurring 8 to 14 days after treatment.

The potential hazards associated with delayed neurotoxicity are twofold:

a. Exposure of occupationally or accidentally exposed individuals who would be affected by high doses for short periods; and
b. Long-term low-level exposure and possible build-up of the toxicant to threshold levels leading to ataxia.

The toxicological hazard associated with such exposure must be considered, not least because it may throw light on the evaluation of the hazards from residues in food.

A key factor in the problem of delayed neurotoxicity is the dose response. Delayed neurotoxicity appears to follow a dose-response relationship and it is therefore possible to estimate a no-effect level following acute or chronic exposure in a susceptible species. With an adequate margin of safety, an acceptable daily intake for man can be allocated with a sufficient degree of assurance as far as pesticide residues in food are concerned.

The toxicological evaluation and possible prevention and treatment of delayed neurotoxicity would benefit considerably from a better understanding of this toxic phenomenon. Further work should be encouraged concerning the possible mechanisms of neurotoxicity, such as the effects on the myelin sheath nerve conduction, motor end-plate function, muscular contraction and spasticity. Studies are also desirable of the mechanisms of the delayed response, including the kinetics of metabolism and tissue distribution.

In addition, further work should be encouraged in the area of delayed neurotoxicity especially with respect to certain areas of concern such as occupational exposure (66).

4.4 Combine effects

Different pesticides and other chemicals are often absorbed simultaneously during occupational use, or in food, by man or animals. It is important that more be learned about their combined toxic effects upon the body. Research should be encouraged on the joint toxic action of pesticides and other chemicals on man and useful animals (67).

4.5 Significance of Interactions

The subject of toxicological interactions between pesticides and between pesticides and other chemicals was extensively reviewed (68) for the purpose of determining whether any such interactions might constitute a consumer hazard. Numerous toxicological interactions can occur between pesticides of the same class, between those of different classes, and between pesticides and drugs.

Detailed consideration is given to interactions between various groups of agents in which pesticides are one or both of the interactants. These groups included organophosphorus with organophosphorus insecticides; organochlorine with organophospharus insecticides and drugs; organophosphorus insecticides with drugs, etc.

At the present levels of pesticide residue intake, the effects that pesticides can have on enzyme systems that metabolize other pesticides or drugs do not appear to present hazards to the consumer and with the continuation of the present criteria for a maximum no-effect level, there should be no need to alter any previous assessment on this account (69).

A subject of particular concern is the possibility that if more than one pesticide is present in a foodstuff the toxic effects may be additive or one pesticide may potentiate the effect of another. The persistent organochlorine insecticides should be considered together in the future and the acceptable daily intake figures for individual compounds be reviewed in the light of the possibility that their toxic effects might be additive or more than additive (70).

5. THE PROCESS OF EVALUATION AND TOXICOLOGICAL DECISIONS

5.1 General Observations

General observations of the process of evaluation and toxicological decisions are the same here as those discussed in the previous chapter in Section 6.1.

5.2. The No-effect Level(s)

In evaluating the toxicological information, the main task is to establish the maximum dose of the compound that could be given over a long period without producing ill effects. In most cases, this is a dose level established in some animal species. For some compounds this level had been determined in man, and such human data, although often covering a relatively short period, naturally have taken precedence. When human data of this type are not available and in the absence of evidence to the contrary, human sensitivity in principle is equated with that of the most sensitive animal species.

It is unfortunate that only crude criteria exist for estimating the mammalian toxicity of many pesticides. A cautious attitude should be adopted towards compounds whose mechanism of action is unknown and which has an effect on life-span or on growth at high doses. Research workers should pay attention to the need for more sensitive criteria for use in this type of work (71).

Each pesticide is toxicologically evaluated on the basis of all the available data on that compound and taking into account relevant data on related compounds and on compounds that give identical or similar metabolites.

It is an essential part of the evaluation to determine the dose levels where no significant toxicological effect is found. These "no-effect" levels in the relevant animal species, and when possible in man, are specified in the comments on each pesticide in published monographs (72).

The identification and selection of a no-effect level from experimental animal data is not an automatic process. In the first place, the interpretation of toxicological data rests on the judgement of the experts, and in the second place, when the toxicological information available on a specific compound is abundant, the selection of a no-effect level from a particular investigation may require time-consuming studies and long consideration.

The no-effect level may be considered to be the daily dose that produces no indication of toxicity in the test animal and it is taken preferably, and when available, from long-term studies in animals of the most appropriate species to permit extrapolation to man.

5.3 Safety Factors and the Problem of Extrapolating
     from Animal Data to Man

Where a maximum no-effect level of dietary intake has been established in a sensitive animal species and where there are no comparable data for man, the animal dose must be taken as a basis for calculating an acceptable daily intake for man. This can be done in several ways. Unfortunately the scientific methods of making this adjustment require an amount of information that is seldom available. Accordingly it is adopted the following empirical method: the maximum no-effec dietary level obtained by animal experiment, expressed in mg/kg body-weight per day, and divided by a "factor," generally 100.

Where the maximum no-effect level of dietary intake in man was known, a smaller factor was used--in certain cases as low as 10 (73).

The magnitude of the safety factor used in establishing acceptable daily intake figures depends on a number of considerations, one of which is the varying susceptibility among species. For this reason adequate biochemical and toxicological data derived from observations in man are of prime importance and could allow the use of considerably smaller safety factor than is the case with data obtained from experimental animals, with obvious consequential advantages (74-76).

A greater margin of safety could also be used where several long-term studies have been reported and where the lowest dosage showed an effect of questionable significance (77). A margin of safety is necessary to allow for differences in sensitivity between the animal species and man, the wide variations in sensitivity among humans beings, and the low number of the experimental animals in comparison with the human population that might be exposed. A thorough discussion of the question of the margin of safety is found in section 6.3 in Chapter I:

In reaffirming the conclusions of a Scientific Group (78), reference is made to the comments stated in the monographs as giving indications of the rationale behind each action taken. It should, however, be emphasized that the magnitude of the margin of safety applied in each individual case is based on the evaluation of all available data. In consideration of any information that gives rise to particular concern, the magnitude of the margin of safety will be increased. Where the data provide an assurance of safety, the magnitude of the safety factor may be decreased. Therefore it is impossible to recommend fixed rules for the margin of safety to be applied in all instances (79).

Recently, the situation regarding safety factors utilized in arriving at ADIs has been further clarified. The establishment of ADIs is not a simple mathematical exercise based on the non-effect level, as the safety factor may vary widely from one compound to another. Although safety factors are determined empirically, they are dependent on the nature of the compound, the amount, nature and quality of toxicological data available, the nature of the toxic effects of the compound, whether an ADI or temporary ADI is established, and the nature of any further data required (206).

5.4 Acceptable Daily Intakes (ADIs) and Other Important Toxicological Decisions

5.4.1 Concept of the ADI and its Rationale

The first aim of the toxicological evaluation is the assessment of the amount of a pesticide to which man can be exposed daily for a lifetime without injury. Of necessity, early views of this amount may be changed and subjected to revision as experience accumulates, particularly after the pesticide has been put into use. When the investigations are completed, it is possible, by the use of scientific judgement, to establish an acceptable daily intake for man, as has been done for certain antimicrobials and antioxidants as stated in the Sixth Report of the Joint FAO/WHO Expert Committee on Food Additives (80).

Based on these considerations, studies should be undertaken to evaluate the evidence, including toxicological and other pertinent data, published and unpublished, on those pesticides known to leave residues in food when used according to good agricultural practices and to issue the conclusions in the form of acceptable daily intake figures, supported by explanations of the basis for each value (81).

Since pesticides are, from their very nature, poisonous to some forms of life, any intake by man in the food may be considered undesirable. For this reason the rate of application of the pesticide to the crop should be as low as possible, and the interval between its last application and the consumption of the crop should be as long as possible so that the residue is reduced to a minimum. Nevertheless,

if pesticides are to be used, as they must be, some ingestion will
occur. It would help in the assessment of any possible hazards arising
from the consumption of these amounts of pesticides if it were known
how much could be consumed daily without risk.

In order to arrive at an acceptable daily intake for man the following
information should be available:

a. The chemical nature of the residue. Pesticides may undergo
chemical changes and are frequently metabolized by the tissues
of the plants and animals which have been treated with them.
Even when a single chemical has been applied, the residue may
consist of a number of derivatives with distinct properties, the
exact nature of which may differ in animals and plants and in
different crops and products;

b. The toxicities of the chemicals forming the residue from acute,
short-term and long-term studies in animals. In addition, knowledge is required on the metabolism, mechanism of action, and
possible carcinogenicity of residue chemicals when consumed;

c. A sufficient knowledge of the effects of these chemicals on man.
Information on this scale is not often available at the present
time, but a daily level of intake having no observable effect on
a sensitive species of animal can be determined. In some cases
this level has been determined for man himself. From this
starting point an acceptable daily intake for man can be proposed
by employing a suitable factor. This is not a blind process and
the nature of the risk is an important consideration. For instance,
although it is conceivable that for a carcinogen dose levels exist
that would not induce cancer, it is considered that the ingestion
of a proven carcinogen as a pesticide residue in human food is
unacceptable.

Similarly, when an acceptable human daily intake of a chemical
has been proposed, the nature of the food bearing the chemical should,
theoretically, be immaterial. Nevertheless, it is considered that
foods such as milk, which is used largely in the diets of babies and
invalids, should be essentially free from pesticide residues.

The amount of data available varies considerably for the different
pesticides. Nevertheless, even when the information about a compound
appears very complete and an acceptable intake is proposed, it must be
realized that the statement that x mg/kg body weight can be eaten every
day for a lifetime without appreciable risk is an expression of opinion.
No matter how carefully the decision is made, it remains an opinion
which carries no guarantee of "absolute" safety. Such a guarantee
would be impossible.

New data or new knowledge can always lead to a re-evaluation of an
acceptable daily intake figure. Values of this nature are always provisional. It is the duty of all who make use of ADI figures to consult
the scientific information on which such figures are based to ensure
that they possess the latest information. It has been decided to propose
only single sets of acceptable daily intake figures. It is, however,
recognized that exceptional situations might arise when owing to a

desperate need for food, the possibility of exceeding these figures, for a strictly limited period of time, would have to be considered. The proposed levels are those that could normally be regarded as acceptable throughout life. They are not set with such precision that they cannot be exceeded for short periods of time.

No guidance is offered to cover unusual circumstances. Each case will have to be decided on its merits by the national authorities responsible. They should take expert advice on the risks to health from excess intake of pesticides and the consequences arising from the loss of the crop.

Since the process of evaluation is a long one, figures of acceptable daily intakes have been recommended for only a limited number of pesticides. The omission of a pesticide from being evaluated does not imply criticism of that pesticide, nor does it suggest that it can be used without restraint (82).

The acceptable daily intake for man has been defined as the daily dosage of a chemical which, if ingested even during an entire lifetime, appears to be without appreciable risk on the basis of all the facts known at the time of the evaluation. 'Without appreciable risk' is taken to mean the practical certainty that injury will not result even after a lifetime of exposure. The acceptable daily intake for man is expressed in milligrams of the chemical, as it appears in the food, per kilogram of body weight (mg/kg/day)(83).

It has been recommended that acceptable daily intake figures should be expressed using only one significant figure. The use of more than one significant figure might be taken to imply a degree of accuracy that cannot be achieved when assessing the hazard from the many factors that influence toxicity (84, 208).

5.4.2 Toxicological Decisions

From the above observations it appears that the ADI figure for man is intended to represent an index of toxicity for pesticide chemicals serving as a basis for assessing the health hazards, if any, of chemicals in the diet. However, the ADI figures can also be considered as one of the important outcomes of the toxicological decisions indicated in the flow diagram in Fig 1 (see Section 6.1, Chapter I). The following terms should be borne in mind when interpreting toxicological experimental results and in formulating toxicological decisions:

ADI. An ADI is allocated only to pesticide chemicals for which the available data include either the results of adequate short-term and long-term toxicological investigations or satisfactory information on the biochemistry and metabolic fate of the compound or both.

Maximum residue limit. A maximum residue limit is defined as the maximum concentration of a pesticide residue that is allowed in or on a food commodity at a specific stage in the harvesting, storage, transport, marketing, or processing of the food, up to the final point of consumption. A maximum residue limit is recommended only when the available residue data so allow, and the toxicity of the pesticide and its metabolites has been adequately assessed.

Extraneous residue limit. An extraneous residue limit is, for a particular commodity, the maximum toxicologically acceptable concentration of a residue unavoidably arising from sources other than the use of a pesticide directly or indirectly for the production of that commodity (85).

Conditional ADI. This decision relates to conditions that have been attached to its use. The practice of the Joint Meeting in adopting conditional ADIs has been different from that of the Joint FAO/WHO Expert Committee on Food Additives in that it implies that there are circumstances in which prpvision is made for special conditions of use and, in general, is established for a pesticide in order to limit its use to those situations where no satisfactory substitutes are available (205).

Temporary ADI and/or maximum residue limit. An ADI or a maximum residue limit may be allocated temporarily, pending the provision of additional information within a stated period of time. This measure implied that the toxicological and/or residue data are adequate to ensure the safety in use of the pesticide during the time for which the temporary clause applied. If the additional data requested do not become available within the stated period, the temporary ADI and/or maximum residue limit may be withdrawn at a future meeting of the committee (86).

No ADI and/or maximum residue limit. This expression is applicable to pesticides for which the available information is not sufficient to establish their safety or when the chemical specifications are not adequate.

Decision postpones. This expression is applicable to cases when no precise information is available.

ADI and/or maximum residue limit withdrawn. This expression relates to cases in which temporary allocations are made but provisions for additional information are not satisfied, or scientific data have shown serious human health hazards.

Guideline levels. These levels are not recommended levels based on adequate assessment of the toxicity of a pesticides, but are sometimes included in the proceedings of the Joint Meeting to assist administering authorities. A guideline level is the maximum concentration of a pesticide residue that might occur after the officially recommended or authorized use of a pesticide for which no acceptable daily intake or temporary acceptable daily intake are established and that need not be exceeded if good practice are followed. It is expressed in milligrams of the residue per kilogram of the food (87).

Tentative negligible daily intake. This term introduced in 1969 (88) was discontinued in 1973 (89).

5.4.3 Administrative Aspects

It has been observed above that the assessment of the toxicity of a pesticide should be thought of as having a dynamic character. This is particularly true with regard to the assessment of the toxicity of those pesticide chemicals which, because of their nature or use, need to be kept under constant review. In addition, new information may become available and may require a revision of previous decisions. In the current terminology, this situation is referred to as "re-evaluation of a pesticide." This task has frequently required the adoption of administrative attitudes designed to ensure the continued awareness of parties interested in generating scientific data and aimed at establishing the safety of pesticide chemicals. The adoption of temporary ADI and/or maximum residue limits, the indication of further work required and/or desirable, and the establishment of deadlines for submission of this work are a few examples of such administrative measures.

Further work required is work that must be done, properly reported and made available within a specific period before acceptable daily intakes for man and/or maximum residue limits can be recommended or confirmed. In certain instances, although acceptable daily intakes have been established, further work has been considered to be essential to remove doubts about the toxicological significance of some experimental observations. Results of the further work required should be made available not later than the specified data, after which the compound will be re-evaluated. The re-evaluation may be done earlier if relevant information should become available.

Further work desirable is work which, when properly reported and made available would be expected to provide additional assurance that acceptable daily intakes for man and recommended maximum residue limits are adequate for the protection of the health of the consumer (90).

5.4.4 Group ADIs

Because some pesticides are closely related chemically and toxicologically, it has been found desirable to establish acceptable daily intakes for groups of such pesticides. This procedure might be extended to include further consideration of the interaction of pesticides belonging to different groups (91).

5.4.5 Evaluation of Metabolites

The acceptable daily intake (ADI) for man applies to the pesticide, together with its metabolites, if the main metabolites present in the residues in the edible portions of farm animals, animal products or plants are identical with the main metabolites in experimental animals. The metabolites must also be present in the same order of magnitude.

If the main metabolites in and on plants and animals are not identical, or if they are identical but not of the same order of magnitude, then the ADI applies only to the original pesticide, and separate studies on the main metabolites in the residues may be necessary for assessment of their of their toxicological properties (92,93).

The major metabolite of a pesticide might not be the most important toxicologically and it might also be necessary to have comparative data on minor metabolites from the chemically related pesticides. Only when such information is available would it be appropriate to consider the extrapolation of toxicological data from one compound to another. On the basis of present knowledge, the only acceptable extrapolation would be when one pesticide is a quantitatively significant metabolite of another pesticide for which adequate toxicological data are available (94).

5.4.6 The Multidisciplinary Approach
to Evaluations

The need for a multidisciplinary approach to the evaluation of the safety of use of pesticides in relation to the occurrence of residues in food is emphasized. A multidisciplinary approach often facilitates the interpretation of the significance of observed effects by providing a range of criteria on which to base judgement of potential toxicity for man (95).

6. SOURCES AND NATURE OF PESTICIDE INFORMATION

6.1 Data necessary to establish ADIs

Toxicological decisions regarding the safety of a substance in general, or its safe limits in particular, belong in the domain of technical and scientific decisions rather than in that of political and administrative ones. These decisions should, therefore, be based solely on technical and scientific knowledge. In turn, political and administrative decisions as to whether a substance should be permitted or limited in its uses are based on the toxicological decisions that have been taken is crucial to the whole process of the toxicological evaluation of a chemical. The quality of the decision will reflect the quality and quantity of the data on which it has been based.

Sources of data on pesticide toxicity are many and varied, and it is unfortunate that very little of the existing scientific information on pesticides is published. This fact has been touched upon on several occasions. For instance, in 1961 it was stated that difficulty in the independent evaluation of the safe use of pesticides was due to the fact that some of them has been brought into use without full publication of the experimental work. It was, therefore, urged that WHO and FAO make every effort to persuade investigators to publish their results in adequate detail (96).

In 1969, during the course of toxicological evaluations, deficiencies were encountered in information, particularly concerning pesticides that had been in use for a long time or which had not been covered by patent rights and which were not actively promoted by commercial interests. With these compounds, it seemed unlikely that the necessary research would be undertaken unless it were initiated by official bodies and supported by public funds (97).

Research promoted by commercial companies, and even that initiated by official bodies, is very often somewhat confidential and consequently may not appear in the published literature. It is not possible to accept and take into account confidential information because it is important that the data on which the assessment is based should be generally available for reference purposes. It is, in fact, the policy of FAO and WHO to make available to bona fide scientists, on request, copies of the unpublished reports quoted in the proceedings of the meeting. It would not be possible to set ADIs or maximum residue limits for pesticides on the basis of abstracts or brief summaries of experimental data. For such purposes a full disclosure of relevant data is necessary (98).

Similar observations were made in 1971 when principles were reaffirmed that the establishment of ADIs and maximum residue limits should be based on all relevant data available at the time of evaluation, that the data used for these purposes should be available to bona fide scientists on request, and that any data used for the establishment of ADIs and maximum residue limits might be quoted in the monographs and reports of the meeting (99).

In commenting on the nature of data and on sources of information, in 1972, it was remarked that the data considered included information from the published literature, government legislation submissions from manufacturers, and reports on research from various sources including manufacturers, universities, agricultural research stations, and toxicological laboratories. Generally, the bulk of the information comes from manufacturers as submitted to regulatory authorities. Information from government agencies concerning toxicology, permitted uses, results of residue surveys and analyses made on commodities moving in commerce, and the need to use a particular pesticide, is valuable but rarely available. On that occasion, the hope was expressed that a suitably qualified organization would take up the task of collecting and collating the toxicological data required, especially on those compounds not sponsored by single manufacturers (100). In 1974 it was again obserbed that in some instances members of the meeting were aware of the existence of information that had not been made available for evaluation. It was, therefore, urged that every effort should be made to seek the cooperation of governments, industry and others to ensure that complete data relating to all compounds reviewed are made available (101).

In 1975, the previous policy of considering unpublished data which can be made available to scientists requesting information or challenging statements made by the meeting was reaffirmed, but the consideration of confidential information was refused (102). Finally, in 1976, the policy was reaffirmed of reviewing relevant published and unpublished information and further all matters relating to the acquisition and availability for data were referred to FAO and WHO, reaffirming that any information that could not be made available for consideration by all members of the meeting would not be taken into account (103).

In re-emphasizing the principles previously laid down for allocating ADIs and temporary ADIs for pesticides, the need for obtaining certain data in order to establish an ADI was reaffirmed. These data include the results of short- and long-term studies on carcinogenicity mutagenicity, reproduction, teratology, observations in man, etc. , as well as information on metabolism, pharmacokinetics, and biochemical effects. Only in exceptional circumstances may an ADI be established in the absence of long-term studies and certain of the studies mentioned above. A temporary ADI may be allocated in cases where the studies needed for a definite evaluation have not been undertaken or are inadequate, but where there is no concern about the safety of the compound that would preclude the daily intake of small quantities for a limited period of time.

In cases where the information is insufficient for the evaluation of the compound, no ADI can be given, but the absence of an ADI does not necessarily mean that the compound is unsafe. In some cases, however, an ADI is not allocated because the data indicated a major toxicological risk (104).

6.2 Published versus Unpublished Toxicological Data

Material published in scientific journals has the advantage of having been considered by editors and referees and of having been open to challenge by other research workers (105). Publication in the scientific examination and criticism and affords the possibility for refutation or confirmation of the results. Consequently, greater weight is usually given to published than to unpublished work. If reports can be submitted only in unpublished form, they must be the result of work supervised by an expert, whose name must be given. Furthermore attention was drawn to the necessity of providing descriptions of experimental techniques that are sufficiently clear to allow checking and assessment of the validity of the results (106).

6.3 Toxicological Data for Pesticides no Longer Covered by Patent

During the course of the toxicological evaluations, deficiencies have been encountered in information particularly concerning pesticides that have been in use for a long time which, for some other reason, are not covered by patent rights and which are not actively promoted by commercial interests. However, with these compounds it seems unlikely that the necessary research will be undertaken unless it is initiated by official bodies and supported by public funds. In particular, it is suggested that FAO should explore the possibilities of obtaining funds for supporting such work on an international basis (107-112).

6.4 The Need for a Reference Publication

In several instances it was recommended that FAO and WHO consider issuing a single volume containing monographs of all pesticides evaluated. This publication would facilitate reference to individual compounds and would be of advantage to those who make use of the information provided (113-116).

6.5 The Need for Pesticide Scientific and Regulatory Information Services

Government offices in many countries receive information on the efficiency and safety of pesticides used in agriculture and food storage and on the persistence and analysis of their residues. This information, which remains unpublished, originates from both governmental and industrial sources. The information provided by industry is often supplied on a confidential basis and cannot receive wider circulation without the firm's consent.

Published scientific and regulatory information on pesticides appears in numerous journals and publications. It is seldom that any government office can keep abreast of these publications. Various journals devoted to providing abstract service cover only a portion of the publications related to pesticides. There is usually a considerable time lag between completion of research and publication of an original paper, and an even further delay before its appearance in the form of an abstract.

This unpublished information is worthy of a wider circulation. National and international groups and government offices responsible for evaluating the efficacy and safe use of pesticides would benefit from it.

It was recognized that both FAO and WHO should provide such a service. It has however, been observed that the scientific aspect of this service should be made more comprehensive, both in coverage and in distribution. For example, the prompt, accurate and wide international exchange of scientific information on efficacy persistence, residue analysis and toxicity of pesticides is essential for their rational use throughout the world.

It was consequently recommended that both FAO and WHO give serious consideration to the establishment of a pesticide scientific and regulatory information service to collect, collate and disseminate published and unpublished information on all aspects of pesticides used in agriculture and food storage. This information should be made generally available to all research and regulatory agencies concerned with the evaluation of pesticides and the formulation of recommendations for their use (117).

6.6 Good Laboratory Practices

Although most of the toxicological data available for the safety evaluation of pesticides are satisfactory, those for a number of compounds are poor or of dubious quality. Other data are derived several years ago and consequently do not comply with the more precise standards and with acceptable laboratory practices. Although all data concerning safety evaluation will be considered valid in normal circumstances, occasions may arise when submitted data may be unacceptable because of low scientific standards or undesirable laboratory practices. Studies from laboratories where such unacceptable standards and practices are known to exist, or to have existed for a definite period, would still be considered, but might require further validation before acceptance. Furthermore, studies conducted in more than one laboratory organization, which support or confirm each other, are likely to have more credibility than uncorroborated data from a single laboratory. Likewise, published data, which provide sufficient information for adequate evaluation and which have been subjected to review, are likely to be more readily accepted than unpublished work (206).

7. USE OF THE ADI FIGURES

7.1 ADI Figures and Toxicity Data

In using the concept of acceptable daily intakes for man in the control of consumer hazard from pesticides, it is not sufficient merely to consult a list of figures. Account must also be taken of the evidence on which the figures are based (118).

7.2 ADI Figures and Maximum Residues Limits

The acceptable daily intake figures are of value as a check to ensure that the recommended maximum residue limits or tolerances are toxicologically acceptable, but in using acceptable daily intake figures in this way some other considerations should be borne in mind.

Addition. ADI figures have been calculated on the assumption that the diet is contaminated by a single chemical residue. In practice foodstuffs frequently contain residues of more than one compound, and additive effects may then occur. As a general safeguard against additive effects, the importance of always keeping the residues to a minimum should be emphasized.

Potentiation. Some organophosphorus compounds potentiate one another's toxic actions so that the effects of administering a mixture are greater than the sum of the effects of their being given alone. Such potentiation may also occur with other pesticides, as well as with other substances and agents to which may is exposed. This may be a serious problem and it should be kept under review.

Genetic differences. The increasing appreciation that genetically determined alterations in the enzymic composition of man can affect his reaction to toxic agents is a further indication that acceptable daily intakes for man should not be applied too rigidly (119).

7.3 ADI Figures and Estimations of Potential
Theoretical Daily Intake of Residues through Food

Having established the acceptable daily intake (ADI) for a pesticide, it becomes paramount that the residue actually ingested with food should not in principle exceed the ADI if the health of the consumer has to be protected. To this end, a relationship between residue limits and acceptable daily intakes for man should be somehow established. This problem is not easily solved as maximum residue limits are proposed on the basis of data on pesticide residues actually obtained or expected on crops which have been grown under good agricultural practices whereas acceptable daily intakes for man are derived from experimental toxicological findings.

In order to establish a relationship between maximum residue limits and acceptable daily intakes for man, potential daily intake calculations have been developed which should represent the theoretical intake of a pesticide calculated on the basis of the maximum residue limits and/or extraneous residue limits and the per caput consumption of the relevant food commodities per day (120). In this respect the World Health Organ-

ization since 1969 has attempted to make estimates of the potential
theoretical intake of pesticide residues using computerized procedures.
A detailed description of this program and the historical impact within
the Joint Meetings and the Codex Committee on Pesticide Residues lies
beyond the scope of this chapter. Table II shows an example of the
layout of the actual calculations and the different variables used in the
study. In examining this table it should be borne in mind that the whole
calculations are based on two important assumptions. Firstly, it is
assumed that the pesticide residue is present in all food items for
which maximum residue limits have been established and secondly,
that the residue is present at the level of the recommended maximum
level. Since neither assumption is correct, the estimated intake is
therefore greater than the actual intake by a factor of usually well
over 10.

Calculations of potential theoretical intakes of the type carried out
by the World Health Organization are generally found useful to show
that further work on the intake of certain pesticides may be unnecessary and to establish priorities in cases where such work is needed.
It would not be advisable, however, to rely upon the results of these
studies alone for quick administrative actions because of their inherent limitations. In effect, among other shortcomings, often no allowance has been made for the effects of processing, storing, and
cooking or the partial disappearance of residues due to lack of adequate
information. Nonetheless, the importance and necessity of generating
data which will serve in extending and perfecting such studies at the
national level cannot be overemphasized if a less pragmatic approach
to the relationship to be established between ADIs and recommended
maximum residue limits is going to be achieved.

The work carried out on the potential theoretical intake of pesticide
residues has been recently reviewed on two occasions, first by a consultation which took place at WHO in 1972 (121) and second by the Third
Joint FAO/WHO Conference on Food Additives and Contaminants (122).
convened at WHO in 1973 on the basis of a recommendation previously
made (123). The conference examined a report (124) outlining the major points of the WHO activities on the computerized calculation on
potential theoretical intakes on chemicals in food. Although it is appreciated that the estimates obtained are not accurate, they provide
indication of the order of magnitude of the potential intake. Clearly
more reliable figures could be obtained only if the average food consumption figures used hitherto could be replaced by more reliable
national food consumption figures supplied by member states. Among
its recommendations, the conference indicates that WHO, in cooperation with FAO, should expand the present work on the computerized
calculation of intakes and include additional countries in the program.
It is to be noted that the emphasis placed by the conference on the need
for reliable food consumption figures may suggest that the previous
models of calculation of potential intakes of pesticide residues might be
profitably adapted to calculation of potential intakes of contaminants
in food, such as mercury and other toxic metals. The need to continue
studies on the potential theoretical daily intake of pesticide residues
has been emphasized regularly (125-132).

TABLE II

POTENTIAL DAILY PESTICIDE RESIDUE INTAKE

ADI : 0.02

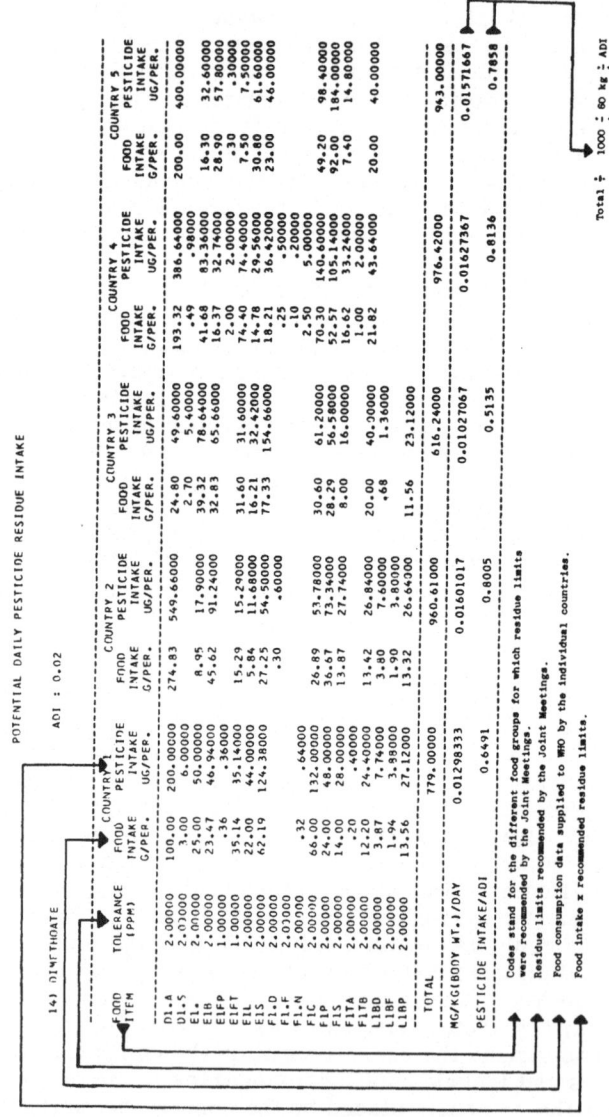

(4) DIMETHOATE

FOOD ITEM	TOLERANCE (PPM)	COUNTRY 1 FOOD INTAKE G/PER.	COUNTRY 1 PESTICIDE INTAKE UG/PER.	COUNTRY 2 FOOD INTAKE G/PER.	COUNTRY 2 PESTICIDE INTAKE UG/PER.	COUNTRY 3 FOOD INTAKE G/PER.	COUNTRY 3 PESTICIDE INTAKE UG/PER.	COUNTRY 4 FOOD INTAKE G/PER.	COUNTRY 4 PESTICIDE INTAKE UG/PER.	COUNTRY 5 FOOD INTAKE G/PER.	COUNTRY 5 PESTICIDE INTAKE UG/PER.
DI-A	2.00000	100.00	200.00000	274.83	549.66000	24.80	49.60000	193.32	386.64000	200.00	400.00000
DI-S	2.00000	3.00	6.00000			2.70	5.40000	.49	.98000		
EI-	2.00000	25.00	50.00000	8.95	17.90000	39.32	78.64000	41.68	83.36000	16.30	32.60000
EIB	2.00000	23.47	46.94000	45.62	91.24000	32.83	65.66000	16.37	32.74000	28.90	57.80000
EIFP	1.00000	.36	.36000					2.00	2.00000	.30	.30000
EIFT	1.00000	35.14	35.14000	15.29	15.29000	31.60	31.60000	74.40	74.40000	7.50	7.50000
EIL	2.00000	22.00	44.00000	5.84	11.68000	16.21	32.42000	14.78	29.56000	30.80	61.60000
EIS	2.00000	62.19	124.38000	27.25	54.50000	77.33	154.66000	18.21	36.42000	23.00	46.00000
FI-D	2.00000							.25	.50000		
FI-F	2.00000							.10	.20000		
FI-N	2.00000	.32	.64000	.30	.60000			2.50	5.00000		
FIJC	2.00000	66.00	132.00000	26.89	53.78000	30.60	61.20000	70.30	140.60000	49.20	98.40000
FIP	2.00000	24.00	48.00000	36.67	73.34000	28.29	56.58000	52.57	105.14000	92.00	184.00000
FIS	2.00000	14.00	28.00000	13.87	27.74000	8.00	16.00000	16.62	33.24000	7.40	14.80000
FITA	2.00000	.20	.40000					1.00	2.00000		
FITB	2.00000	12.20	24.40000	13.42	26.84000	20.00	40.00000	21.82	43.64000	20.00	40.00000
LIBD	2.00000	3.87	7.74000	3.80	7.60000	.68	1.36000				
LIBF	2.00000	1.94	3.88000	1.90	3.80000						
LIBP	2.00000	13.56	27.12000	13.32	26.64000	11.56	23.12000				
TOTAL			779.00000		960.61000		616.24000		976.42000		943.00000
MG/KG(BODY WT.)/DAY			0.01298333		0.01601017		0.01027067		0.01627367		0.01571667
PESTICIDE INTAKE/ADI			0.6491		0.8005		0.5135		0.8136		0.7858

Total ÷ 1000 ÷ 60 kg ÷ ADI

Codes stand for the different food groups for which residue limits were recommended by the Joint Meetings.

Residue limits recommended by the Joint Meetings.

Food consumption data supplied to WHO by the individual countries.

Food intake x recommended residue limits.

8. INTERNATIONALLY RECOMMENDED
MAXIMUM RESIDUE LIMITS FOR PESTICIDES

The FAO members of the Joint Meeting are responsible mainly for establishing and recommending maximum residue limits for pesticides and the Codex Committee on Pesticide Residues is responsible for proposing international maximum residue limits for the consideration of the Joint FAO/WHO Codex Alimentarius Commission. In endorsing provisions for maximum residue limits, the Codex Committee takes into account the toxicological evaluations and the maximum residue limits recommended by the Joint Meeting.

At first sight and in principle this system may be thought to be conducive to the formation of two different sets of figures representing internationally recommended maximum residue limits since the Codex Committee on Pesticide Residues may or may not accept the figures recommended by the Joint Meeting. In practice this has very seldom occurred, either because the harmonization methodology adopted by the Codex Committee over the years has become more and more oriented towards scientific information or because of the continuous and effective feedback between the two groups.

8.1 Statement of the Problem

In Appendix V of the report of the first session of the Codex Committee on Pesticide Residues in 1966, a chapter was included which outlines basic principles for the adoption of internationally recommended maximum residue limits for pesticides and procedures for determining such limits.

Some of the important points are summarized below:

At the present time, recourse must be made to pesticides both in the production of crops and to protect them from damage once they have been harvested. While some of the chemicals used for this purpose do not contaminate the final crop, others, even when used according to good agricultural practices, leave residues in food at the time of consumption. In this connection the expression "residues" applies to residues of the chemical compounds themselves and to metabolites, breakdown products or other chemical substances derived from them. Pesticides are also used in the protection of livestock. Residues from this use and from animal feed treated with pesticides may also be present in foodstuffs of animal origin. The human diet may therefore contain pesticide residues from various sources.

Residues of pesticides in unprocessed foodstuffs usually result in smaller residues at the time when foods from them are consumed. When proposing tolerances for residues in foodstuffs, it is necessary to indicate the point at which the tolerances are valid and enforceable. For international trade in grain and grain products it is proposed that the tolerances be applicable at the point of entry of the commodity into the importing country. Because many commodities such as raw grain are not consumed in their imported state but are further processed with a resultant reduction in residue content, the tolerance of residues at the point of entry may sometimes exceed the level that would be acceptable at the time of consumption.

The detection of the presence of a pesticide residue depends on the sensitivity and the specificity of the analytical method. When investigations into the good agricultural practice in the use of a pesticide have established that there need be no residue, it may be possible and useful in some cases to establish a tolerance as a protection against misuse of the material. When this is done the tolerance should be at the minimum level that can be determined by an internationally adopted analytical method. Background residues must be taken into account when setting such a tolerance.

Pesticides whose residues are known to disappear or to be converted into harmless substances during storage, processing, or cooking of certain treated commodities may be exempted from the requirement of pesticide tolerance on those commodities.

The establishment of residue tolerances for use in a world-wide basis requires careful consideration of many factors by many national and international groups. It must be recognized that there are differences in legally established or accepted tolerances for the same pesticide in different countries. The acceptance of international tolerances under the Codex Alimentarius Commission should help to adjust differences in tolerance which have arisen as a result of individual national action on widely varying principals.

No doubt it will take several years to review and to take action upon all the pesticides currently in use. Accordingly, the fact that a tolerance or an exemption from a tolerance has not been established should not be interpreted as indicating that the pesticide is not acceptable for use. On the other hand, a decision to allot a tolerance to a pesticide residue in a particular crop indicates tacit recognition of the use of the pesticide on that crop at least to the limits of the tolerance permitted. If the residue in a particular crop should be reduced to the absolute minimum, a tolerance should be set at the level which is the minimum that can be determined by internationally adopted analytical methods.

The producer, under the guidance of the appropriate advisory agency, should apply the pesticide in a way, at a concentration, at intervals and at a period before harvest that keeps the residue as low as possible. This approach requires a thorough biological knowledge of the pest or disease under the prevailing regional and climatic conditions and of the response to pesticides under these conditions.

Differences in agricultural practice, in soils and climates, in pest and disease problems, and in the application of biological and chemical knowledge result in differences in residues of pesticides in products from different countries. National tolerances based solely on the actual pesticide residues found in crops in a particular locality can therefore sometimes be a handicap to international trade in foodstuffs which, although not necessarily carrying harmful residues, may have them in excess of tolerances in force in receiving countries. This difficulty can be dealt with in two ways. Either the producing country can control the use of the pesticide more effectively in crops destined for international commerce, or the importing country can accept imported foodstuffs containing residues higher than its own national tolerances would permit.

This position leads to a requirement to revalue national tolerance levels, which, in turn, necessitates international agreement on the principles for establishing residue tolerances. As a first step, a country proposing a tolerance for a residue of a particular chemical on a crop it wishes to export or import could submit sufficient evidence of the actual residues together with a justification or comments on their magnitude. It would then expect the importing or exporting country to re-examine its tolerance levels or agricultural practices in the light of the new information supplied. This could lead to the reconsideration of the figures for national tolerances. The establishment of an international tolerance based on public health needs is the logical conclusion of such a process (133).

8.2 Definitions and Glossaries

While the problem related to the need for internationally adopted maximum residue limits for pesticides has been relatively easily defined, the procedure for setting these limits has been the object of continuous unravelling developments, as testified by the many attempted definitions and glossaries of terms which are found in the numerous documents resulting from the activities of the Joint Meeting and the Codex Committee on Pesticide Residues. A detailed analysis of these developments would go far beyond the scope of this chapter. However, a few examples are cited in order to demonstrate the complexity of the problem.

The Joint Meeting in 1963 wished to re-emphasize the fundamental differences which exist between acceptable daily intake figures and figures for "tolerances." Only acceptable daily intakes, being based entirely on toxicological evidence, can be accorded an international scientific agreement. A "tolerance" is the smallest residue consistent with the control of the pest, but to be toxicologically acceptable it mu.t not exceed the permissible levels, tolerances, etc. , that were proposed and defined (135). Later previously accepted terms were changed, dropped, or their conceptual content modified. The growth, both in number and complexity, of terminology related to pesticide residues was such that the Joint Meeting felt the need to condense adopted terms into a glossary (136). An ad hoc Drafting Group on Principles for Establishing and Enforcing Pesticide Tolerances, which met in Ottawa in 1969, agreed that the definitions contained in this glossary could be improved (137). This glossary was later revised (138) and a further revision was suggested (139) and finally carried out (140). Definitions of terms used by the Codex Committee on Pesticide Residues can also be found in reports they published (141, 142).

The search for a relatively easy mathematical formula for establishing internationally recommended figures for "tolerances" had tempted from the very outset both the Joint Meeting and the Codex Committee. This rather simple approach to a complex problem is suggested by the calculation reported (143) and by the formula reported in subsequent publications (144, 145).

It soon became apparent, however, that no single formula could approach for estimating "tolerances" was subsequently rejected by the

Joint Meeting when it was agreed that initial proposals for "tolerances" should be made on the basis of residues that result when pesticides are used in accordance with good agricultural practice (146, 147).

It should be noted that the existing international maximum residue limits recommended by the Joint Meeting have been based on the above procedure. It is, however, unfortunate that the early attempts to use mathematical formulae probably contributed to the proliferation of formulae still prevalent today in certain groups in charge of establishing tolerances for pesticides at a national level.

8.3 Current Procedures and Terminology

The current procedures for determining maximum residue limits were outlined in detail by the Joint Meeting in 1972 (147) and are described below:

Thorough studies are performed on published literature, government legislation, submissions from manufacturers, and reports on research from various sources, including manufacturers, universities, and agricultural research stations. Generally the bulk of the information from government agencies concerning permitted uses, results of residue surveys and analyses made on commodities moving in commerce, and the need to use a particular pesticide is valuable but rarely available.

Only residue data from trials carried out in conformity with registered or approved use patterns are employed as a basis for recommendations. However, attention is paid to the effect on residue levels of the number of applications, application rates, and the interval between final application and harvest.

Considerable attention is paid to the question of metabolites, degradation products, and impurities that might appear as residues in plant or animal products and the significance of each is considered. Where such substances appear as significant residues at or after harvest, appropriate mention is made in the recommendations.

Where available, data on disappearance during storage, processing, and cooking are considered and reference is made in the monographs. However, since it is necessary to base the proposals on levels to be found in raw agricultural products, the tolerance levels normally recommended are much higher than those of the residues actually present in the prepared food eaten by the consumer.

To guide regulatory authorities in their examination of commodities moving in trade at some stage later than harvest, information on the rate of reduction during storage is provided, where this has been determined. Likewise, information that indicates the location of the residue on or in the commodity (on skin, shell, leaves, husks, or in fat, meat, juice, pulp, etc.) is provided when available.

The minimum interval permitted between the last application and harvest varies considerably from country to country. This does not necessarily mean that the residue level at harvest varies to the same degree. The practice of the Joint Meeting is to select results reflecting the most generally approved interval, unless there are special circumstances that indicate that some other interval should be considered.

The uses of any compound against a pest on a particular crop vary considerably from region to region, owing to differences in ecology, climate, and cultural practices. The residue levels at harvest consequently vary over a range.

The expert group considers the available information on agricultural practices and makes an effort to base recommendations only on normal conditions in the regions where there is a need to use the pesticide. If, in the opinion of the experts, the requirements in certain regions justify multiple applications or applications shortly before harvest, consideration is given to these needs. It would not be possible to recommend significantly lower levels without seriously interfering with pest control practices. Residue data resulting from an exceptional need to use high application rates immediately before harvest are not generally used as a basis for recommendations.

Recent definitions by the Joint Meeting (148) relate to definitions of maximum residue limit, temporary maximum residue limit, extraneous residue limit and guideline level. These definitions are given below:

A maximum residue limit is the maximum concentration of a pesticide residue resulting from the use of a pesticide according to good agricultural practice directly or indirectly for the production and/or protection of the commodity for which the limit is recommended. The maximum residue limit should be legally recognized. It is expressed in milligrams of the residue per kilogram of the commodity. The expression "maximum residue limit" replaces the formerly used "tolerance" in accordance with the practice initiated by the 1972 Joint Meeting.

A temporary maximum residue limit is a maximum residue limit established for a specified, limited period. The expression "temporary maximum residue limit" replaces the formerly used "temporary tolerance" in accordance with the practice initiated by the 1972 Joint Meeting.

A temporary maximum residue limit is proposed under either of the following conditions:

a. When only a temporary or conditional acceptable daily intake has been established for the pesticide concerned; or
b. When, although an acceptable daily intake has been established, the residue data are inadequate for firm maximum residue recommendations.

Residues for which data are inadequate include those for which information or losses of residue during storage, handling and preparation is inadequate and for which calculations based on the inadequate figures indicate that the potential daily intake could be exceeded. In cases of this kind temporary maximum residue limits are recommended only after the Joint Meeting has considered information on the actual occurrence of residues in food, obtained from total diet and similar studies, and after it is satisfied that the potential daily intake is not likely to be exceeded. The information considered includes the results from subjective and/or from objective sampling, including total diet studies, in various countries and particularly in places where pesticides are most widely used. Temporary maximum residue limits will be reviewed no later than the first meeting following the specified date.

An extraneous residue limit is, for a particular commodity, the maximum toxicologically acceptable concentration of a residue unavoidably arising from sources other than the use of a pesticide directly or indirectly for the production of that commodity. The extraneous residue limit should be legally recognized. Residues in food of animal origin arising from residues in animal feed derived from activities that are controllable by farming practices are covered by "maximum residue limits." The term "practical residue limits" which has led to much confusion has been abandoned.

A guideline level is the maximum concentration of a pesticide residue that might occur after the officially recommended or authorized us use of a pesticide for which no acceptable daily intake or temporary acceptable daily intake is established and that need not be exceeded if good practices are followed. It is expressed in milligrams of the residue per kilogram of the food.

Other current aspects relate to the ways of expressing residue limits. In this respect the Joint Meeting supported the adoption of metric units and urged that recommendations of residue levels should be expressed in mg/kg (149). In addition, it discussed the significance of proposing residue limits based on geometrical rather than arithmetical progression (150).

9. CRITERIA FOR TOXICOLOGICAL EVALUATION OF SOME REPRESENTATIVE CLASSES OF PESTICIDE CHEMICALS

9.1 Fumigants

The meeting decided that a somewhat different approach was needed in considering fumigants. To make the report as complete and as useful as possible, it has been decided to evaluate the possible consumer hazards arising from all the uses of fumigants on food but not those arising from other uses of these substances, e. g. as soil fumigants.

Fumigants for food form a fairly well-defined group of substances which have remained unaltered in number and composition for many years. These substances have been developed as fumigants and have become accepted as suitable for that purpose for three reasons: a. they are effective against the pest; b. although many of them are highly toxic, it has been possible to derive ways of using them safely; and c. it has been considered in the past that use of these fumigants would not lead to a consumer hazard provided the operators adhered to good practice in regard to type of crop, dosage, method of application and subsequent treatment of the crop (aeration, milling, baking, etc.). The meeting did not concern itself with the possible hazards that these fumigants might offer to their users.

Fumigants could give rise to a consumer hazard in several ways:

a. The fumigants might persist on the food chemically unchanged as a residue which would be consumed;

b. The fumigant might persist on the food chemically unchanged as a residue different in composition from the fumigant itself which would also persist and might finally be consumed;

c. The fumigant might interact chemically with the food to form a new substance which might also persist as a residue;

d. The fumigant might interact chemically with the food in such a way as to affect its nutritional value.

If a fumigant when used according to good practice had none of these actions, it could not present a consumer hazard and its use would be acceptable. For the assessment of the dangers that might arise from a fumigant which did have one or more of these actions, the concepts of "acceptable daily intakes" might be useful in the cases when there was a residue of either the unchanged fumigant, its decomposition products, or the chemical substances it had formed with the food. Knowledge of the "acceptable daily intakes" of these substances would be useful in assessing consumer hazards that might arise from the use of the fumigant, particularly under conditions of abnormal pest infestation when the dose might have to be increased or the treatment repeated.

Where the fumigant had a deleterious effect on the nutritive value of the foodstuff, one would have to know which nutrient in the food had been affected, what alternative sources of that nutrient were present in the diet, the importance of the fumigated food as a source of that nutrient were present in the diet, and the importance of the fumigated food as a source of that nutrient to the population at risk. The suitability of the fumigant would be judged on the answers to these questions and the decision might differ in different areas.

It is realized that for most fumigants little information is available on residues left in the various items of food treated. Further, the chemical reactions that might take place between the fumigants and components such as aminoacids or vitamins in the food have been insufficiently investigated. This situation is very unsatisfactory and it is urgently recommended that governments initiate research to solve the problems connected with the fumigation of food. In view of the unsatisfactory situation it is urged that, for the safety of both user and consumer, all fumigants should be used in accordance with good practices, paying particular attention to the choice of the food to be treated, subsequent aeration of the food, and the removal of any material used to generate the fumigant.

An acceptable daily intake for the residue of the unchanged fumigant was established in only one case, that of hydrogen cyanide. The residue of inorganic bromide from the use of ethylene dibromide is thought to be unlikely to make any significant contribution to the total bromide content of the diet. The use of methyl bromide can lead to higher residues of inorganic bromide. It is considered that the possible risk from these residues could be assessed, if need be, on the basis that the total daily intake of this ion from all sources should not exceed 1 mg of Br per kg body-weight per day.

Carbon tetrachloride and ethylene dibromide are not considered to lead to a consumer hazard provided that none of the unchanged fumigant

reached the consumer. It is also thought that ethylene dichloride should
be used as a fumigant under conditions that will result in the lowest
possible residues in the food consumed.

For methyl bromide, ethylene oxide, acrylonitrile and phosphine,
there is insufficient toxicological evidence available to evaluate the
significance of any residues of the unchanged fumigants. Since phosphine is often generated in grain from aluminium phosphide it is considered that crops treated with this substance should be freed of residues of the powder before they reached the consumer.

Acceptable daily intakes could not be determined for carbon disul-
fide or chloropicrin and a large amount of work will be necessary on
the nature and amount of the residues and the interaction of the fumigants with the treated food, in addition to long-term toxicological studies, if the use of these fumigants is to be continued. These remarks do
not apply to the use of chloropicrin as a warning agent (151).

Extensive data on the effects of inhalation of fumigants and in some
cases on their fate in the body are generally available in experimental
animals and man. These data, which have been used in establishing
maximum permissible concentrations for occupational exposure as time-
weighted averages, could also be adapted to provide a no-effect level
for oral administration. This evaluation should take into account the
possibilities that continuous ingestion may occur and that certain groups
of consumers (e. g. , children, pregnant women, old people, individuals
with illness or impaired physiological functions) may be more sensitive
than the adult workers who are generally submitted to medical control.
To use these data for this purpose, precise information is needed on
the extent of absorption of each fumigant through the lungs, possibly
through the skin and by oral route when animals are exposed to the
vapor. It should also be recognized that for some fumigants, the fate
in the body may be different with various routes of absorption. For
these reasons some oral feeding studies of at least 90 day duration are
required. Such studies have been undertaken in only very few cases
(152).

Data were reviewed pertaining to the occurrence of residues from
the use of methyl bromide and ethylene dibromide in foods and agreed
that there would be a continuing need to consider residues of bromine
occurring as inorganic bromide. Nevertheless, the occurrence of residues of the fumigants in unreacted form in certain foods has been reported, and some of the older data on this subject do not clearly differentiate residues in organic form from those occurring in the food
as inorganic bromide. It was therefore decided to review the position
of residues of these two fumigants, together with those from carbon
tetrachloride, ethylene dichloride and ethylene oxide, when results
should be available following the use of recently developed sensitive
analytical methods for measuring residues of these compounds. However, it is recommended that no further consideration be given to
trichloroethylene at present because the compound is rarely used as a
fumigant and no residues of it have been found in food commodities
moving in commerce (153).

The fumigants are characterized by their high volatility relative to
most other types of pesticide. The total residue at the end of the fumi-

gation period consists of "physically held" (sorbed) unchanged fumigant and also the products of any chemical reaction between sorbed fumigant and the food. The process of physical uptake is reversible and during subsequent storage, handling and processing of the food the physically sorbed fumigant tends to disappear by volatilization and diffusion away from the food, and possibly also by further chemical reaction with the food.

It has previously been generally accepted that after use in accordance with good practice no significant residue of the unchanged fumigant reaches the consumer and some countries setting national tolerances for pesticide residues have exempted a number of these fumigant compounds from the requirement for establishment of a tolerance.

More sensitive and more selective methods of fumigant residue analysis have recently been developed and these have been used to follow changes in the amounts of unchanged fumigant in certain foods after fumigation. The results confirm that the amount of the residual unchanged fumigant continues to decline during storage handling or processing, but indicate that in some circumstances small amounts may still be detectable in food when offered for consumption. The desirability of reducing such residues to a minimum in food is stressed by the adoption of good practice in handling the food after fumigation.

A special difficulty arises in the application of tolerances at the point of entry of a commodity into a country. Since fumigation is frequently undertaken immediately before shipping, or even during transit in ships' holds or containers, the amounts of volatile or reactive residues will be changing rapidly at the time of discharge. It has therefore been specified that such produce should not be sampled for analysis until the commodity has been discharged, ventilated or freely exposed to the air for a period of at least 24 hours after the end of treatment (154).

9.2 Organohalogenated Compounds

9.2.1 Effects on the Liver (see also Section 4.1)

Organochlorine pesticides have been used extensively and have proved efficacious. Many have been shown to be persistent and comulative in the animal and human body. In addition, there is evidence that even in low doses they have an effect on the liver. During the past few years, evidence has become available that these compounds stimulate the activity of microsomal enzymes in the liver cells. These enzymes may affect the metabolism of other compounds. The toxicological significance of these changes is difficult to interpret. It was strongly recommended that WHO should promote the development of toxicological studies on these compounds to resolve any doubts that may still remain about their safety to consumers (155, 156). WHO should also examine the interpretation given to the effects of pesticides on microsomal enzymes and should also study certain related subjects (157).

9.2.2 Environmental Contamination

Noting that the occurrence of unintentional residues in a number of food items and animal feedstuffs is partly a result of environmental contamination, it was recommended that efforts be made to discover the sources of such contamination and, where possible, to eliminate them, in order to reduce the background level of pesticide residues. Two possible sources are the appearance of pesticides in animal feedstuffs and the widespread use of aerosol dispensers, pressurized or hand sprayers, hand vaporizers, etc. , in homes, restaurants and other places where food is prepared for sale or consumption. That elimination of these sources, as far as practicable, would reduce the background level of pesticide residues is evidenced by some recent surveys of the levels of organochlorine insecticides in the human body.

Concern is also expressed over the extent of use of certain persistent pesticides. This results in contamination of the environment by these substances and it is suggested replacing them, wherever possible, by pesticides whose residues are less undesirable toxicologically (158).

The understandable concern over the contamination of the environment from certain uses of persistent pesticides is noted, and recommendations are made with respect to DDT and seed treatment chemicals (159).

9.2.3 DDT

Current concern over the potential hazard from DDT is based on a. its ubiquity, b. its persistence in the environment and the effect on some wildlife, c. its retention in living organisms, d. its capacity to be transferred to and to be retained in the fetus, and e. the existence of some experimental evidence of its capacity to induce tumors in experimental animals. The relevance to human health of this information, particularly on the last aspect, has been considered.

Although the available experimental data do not provide sufficient information to allow a definite evaluation of the potential carcinogenicity of DDT, they do strongly indicate that DDT ought to be extensively tested. A definite decision on the potential hazard of DDT to man could not be taken at this time. However, because the hazard to man from DDT has not been ruled out, it is emphasized that uses of DDT should be limited to those situations where there were no satisfactory substitutes. While the desirability of introducing alternative compounds and alternative methods of control is stressed, recognition is given to the vital role that DDT and some other organochlorine pesticides play in the food production and protection programs of many countries because of its low cost, user safety, lack of suitable substitutes and safety in its storage and transport. For example, it is estimated that DDT and other organochlorine compounds represent considerably more than half the total insecticides used in the argiculture of developing countries. Maintenance, development and any expansion of the essential protection of food and fiber by alternative chemicals would be beyond the financial resources of many countries at the present time and could involve the introduction of new risks for which users and others are not yet prepared. Indeed, in terms of food supply and welfare of expanding populations, the continuing and controlled use of DDT and some other organochlorine pesticides is essential in the present state of knowledge.

It is noted that total diet studies carried out in a few countries where DDT was sidely used had revealed that the intakes of DDT and its metabolites are well below the ADI established. In addition, the replacement of persistent organochlorine insecticides by alternatives is being increasingly dictated by problems of pest resistance. In several countries, use patterns and scales of use of DDT are under review, with likely reductions in residue levels in many food crops (160).

Following the publication of a report indicating that long-term exposure of several generations of mice to DDT resulted in an increasing incidence of tumors at various sites in later generations, the ADI of DDT was changed to a "conditional ADI" and lowered from 0.01 mg/kg body-weight to 0.005 mg/kg (8).

Having reviewed an interim publication from the authors of the report, in 1967 it has already been recommended that the International Agency for Research on Cancer (IARC) initiate extensive testing of the possible carcinogenicity of DDT. Results of these studies, carried out in parallel at the IARC laboratory in Lyon, France, and the National Institute for the Study and Therapy of Tumours in Milan, Italy, showed that exposure of two strains of mice to the highest dose level of DDT used (250 mg of DDT per kg of animal diet, equivalent to a daily intake of 37.5 mg per kg of body-weight) resulted in an increased incidence of parenchymal liver cell tumors, some of which were malignant. At this high level of exposure, the tumor incidence was increased in both sexes and there was a significant shortening of the life span. At the lowest dose level (2 mg of DDT per kg of animal diet, equivalent to a daily intake of 0.3 mg per kg of body-weight) an increased incidence of liver tumors was observed in the males of one strain only. Results from tests on these two strains of mice did not confirm the occurrence of tumors at multiple sites, nor was there any increase in incidence of tumors at any site from the first generation to the second. It was noted that the lowest dose tested in the mice was more than 100 times the average daily intake for man.

After examining the new information, it was felt that experts were not yet in a position to evaluate the nature and implication of all the data available. It was considered, however, that the "conditional ADI" of 0.005 mg per kg of body-weight as defined and established in 1969 should be maintained, and that this conditional ADI should be reconsidered when further results from current and additional studies, in particular comparative metabolic and epidemiological studies, become available. Moreover, it was recognized that there are particular circumstances where the benefits to man arising from the proper use of DDT outweigh the possible risk from exposure (161).

The attention of toxicologists has been focused during recent years on the tumorigenic action of DDT on mouse liver, and this question has been under constant scrutiny. Data were presented that demonstrated that mice ingesting 36 mg of DDT per kg of body-weight in their feed for 15 weeks developed hepatomas that did not regress. However, no

tumors have thus been produced in any other species tested, * e. g. ,
rats and hamsters. Furthermore, the limited epidemiological data
available give no indication that DDT might be a human carcinogen. A
number of people have had intermittent heavy exposure to DDT over a
period of some 30 years, which should be sufficient time to produce
and observe any increased tumor incidence that might have occurred.
There is an urgent need for new epidemiological data that would permit an evaluation of the implications of the results obtained in mice
(162).

9.2.4 Hexachlorobenzene (HCB)

In 1969, on the basis of the results of a 13 week feeding study in
rats in which no adverse effects were detected at a daily dosage of
1.25 mg/kg, a "tentative negligible daily intake" of 0-0.0006 mg/kg
bw was estimated, and it was indicated that before an ADI could be
established several toxicological studies would be required. In 1973,
it was decided that the term "tentative negligible daily intake" should
not be used.

Since 1969 no further work relevant to estimating an ADI has become available. It is known, however, that several laboratories are
currently engaged in research that might provide a reasonable basis
for the safety evaluation of HCB, and it was urged that these data
should be obtained for future consideration.

It is recognized that HCB residues in foods also arise from sources
other than its proper use as a fungicide (e. g. , industrial wastes from
chlorination processes and contamination of other chlorinated pesticides). Because of this, it will not be sufficient to attempt to control
exposure merely by controlling the use of HCB as a fungicide. Not-
withstanding the fact that residues of HCB stem less from its use as
a pesticide than from other sources, the recommendation made in 1969
that a suitable substitute for HCB as a seed fungicide should be sought
was reaffirmed. In addition, it is recommended that efforts should be
made to reduce the level of HCB as an impurity in other pesticides.
A specific recommendation to this effect is made in the case of quinto-
zene.

On the assumption that there is a level of HCB below which no significant toxicological effects can be expected, it is felt possible to give
some provisional guidance. A daily intake of 0.0006 mg/kg is considerably below any dosage rate known to be harmful, and it is recommended that this value should be used as a guide for setting upper limits
for residues until it is possible to establish an ADI based on the results
of comprehensive toxicological studies. Concern is expressed that some
effects attributed to HCB might be due to impurities in the test samples.

*Note of the author: A recent study by oral administration claims DDT
  has having produced carcinogenic effects in rats (see Int. J. Cancer,
  19, 179-185, 1977).

It is noted that there is an increasing number of reports of HCB residues in foods, feeds and human tissues. Since the sources of these residues are known to include disposal of industrial and municipal wastes, contamination of HCB of other chlorinated pesticides, the approved use of HCB as a seed-dressing, and misuse of HCB-treated seeds in animal feeds it is urged that:

a. Support should be given to an international monitoring program for detecting the sources and extend of contamination;
b. The presence of HCB as an impurity in other pesticides should be monitored and minimized;
c. The recommendations for use of HCB as a seed dressing (163) be carefully adhered to; and
d. HCB should be used only as a seed dressing and only when suitable substitute is available.

In view of the potential toxicity of hexachlorobenzene and the lack of adequate toxicological data to assess its safety, WHO and FAO should promote and where necessary coordinate research needed on this seed-dressing fungicide (164).

Recently published reports on tests for mutagenic and teratogenic action, studies of biochemical effects, histopathological studies, tissue disposition studies and reproduction studies were examined. Although none of these are long-term studies, the results reported permit a reaffirmation of the previously suggested value of 0.0006 mg per kg of body-weight (165, 166) as a guide for setting upper limits for residues. Since the results of a long-term feeding and carcinogenesis study known to be in progress are not yet available, the full evaluation for an ADI is deferred, but it is allocated a value of 0.0006 mg per kg body-weight as a conditional ADI.

Because of the persistent nature of HCB and its widespread occurrence in the environment, it must be recognized that even if all sources of emission could be stopped, some food contamination with HCB will continue for many years (167).

9.2.5 Body Burden of Halogenorganic Compounds

Concern is expressed at the total environmental concentration and the human body burden of halogenorganic chemicals and their possible chemical and biological interactions. These substances at relatively high dosage are known to produce hypertrophy of the liver cells, proliferation of the endoplasmic reticulum and induction of the hepatic microsomal enzymes in many mammalian species. Although in many circumstances, single organochlorine chemicals may or may not present a hazard to man in combination and in the presence of other chemicals, they could present a greater hazard because of the high overall dosage or chemical or biological interactions.

It has already been recommended that the significance and interrelationship of these biological phenomena should be investigated with reference to the health hazards of certain pesticides for man (210, 211).

It is, therefore, proposed that the WHO should convene a special meeting to consider this phenomenon and the associated potential hazards to human health (206).

9.3 Organomercurial Compounds

Attention is drawn to the statement of the FAO/WHO Expert Committee on Food Additives (168) that "the use of alkyl or aryl mercury fungicides as seed-treating agents should be discouraged and the Committee recommends that the use of mercury compounds in agriculture be reviewed, in the light of this report, by the FAO Working Party of Experts on Pesticide Residues and the WHO Expert Committee on Pesticide Residues."

A wide range of organomercury compounds are used in agriculture. These fall into three main classes: alkyl, alkoxy-alkyl and aryl compounds. The main usage of these compounds is for the treatment of cereal and other seeds before sowing. Other applications include the treatment of rice plants at early stages of growth and of fruit trees before flowering. The latter have since become less frequent and at present seed dressings are the only significant agricultural usage.

Although it is not possible to conduct a detailed enquiry into the various reasons for treating seeds with fungicides or into the efficacy of possible replacements, it is known that mercury dressings are needed in certain situations and against particular plant diseases. Satisfactory alternatives are not currently available. It is recognized that at least a small proportion of the more volatile alkylmercury compounds is much greater than that of arylmercury ones and treatment levels increase very considerably according to whether alkylmercury, alkoxy-alkylmercury or arylmercury compounds are used.

Organomercury fungicides, particularly the alkylmercury compounds, have been implicated in incidents of poisoning, including fatal poisoning in man. The most serious incidents have been due to the consumption of treated seed accidentally or improperly diverted from its intended use for sowing. Some evidence is also available concerning the extent to which seed dressings contribute to the amount of mercury in the environment. Bearing in mind that arylmercury and other forms of mercury can be transformed into alkylmercury (principally methylmercury) compounds by certain organisms in nature, the evidence does not clearly differentiate between the potential contributions of arylmercury and alkylmercury compounds and that of naturally occurring inorganic mercury.

However, it is clear that the amount of mercury used in agriculture represents only a small proportion of the total released into the environment from all sources, e.g., in the USA, agricultural uses account for only some 2% of the release of mercury. The amount of mercury added to soil by seed dressings is usually small in comparison with the normal levels of mercury in the soil. There is very little likelihood of mercury from treated seeds finding its way into streams or other water, except as a result of gross carelessness.

In view of the serious cases of human poisoning by mercury fungicides and the difficulty of preventing dressed seed from being diverted
for consumption by man or animals, especially in certain countries,
it was recommended that further study should be given to the question
of replacing them, wherever possible, by compounds less likely to
produce such poisoning incidents (169).

9.4 Organophosphorus Compounds

9.4.1 Cholinesterase Inhibition

The major criterium for evaluation of some OP compounds and carbamates is the in vivo inhibition of ChE and aliesterase (171).
In discussing on which elements an establishment of acceptable
daily intake should be based, it is observed that, in the past, ADIs
have occasionally been established for pesticides for which the results
of long-term studies in animals were not available. The scientific
literature contains an increased number of examples of substances
that have been presumed to be safe solely on the basis of chemical,
metabolic, and short-term toxicological information, but that have
subsequently been shown to exhibit toxic effects in long-term studies
in laboratory animals. It is therefore agreed that only in exceptional
circumstances should ADIs be established in the absence of satisfactory data from long-term animal studies. However, for some OP
pesticides it may still be logical to base ADIs on data from adequate
short-term in vivo studies of anti-ChE activity, since such activity is
the most sensitive criterion of effect for these compounds. Nevertheless, data from long-term experiments are usually required to provide assurance of the safety of moieties of molecules other than those
responsible for the anti-ChE activity (172).
For animals exposed to OP compounds that inhibit ChE, depression
of ChE activity in plasma, erythrocytes, and various other tissues is
usually the most sensitive measure of toxicity. However, a few organophosphorus (OP) compounds with low acute toxicity and certain carbamates produce reversible inhibition of ChE. Measurement of depression of ChE activity in blood or tissues may then be unreliable as an
indicator of potential toxicity.
Because of anti-ChE effect of certain carbamates is reversible and
because many of them have only short half-lives, information on
plasma concentrations and biological half-lives of such compounds is
required. Such information is needed to elucidate discrepancies between signs of cholinergic stimulation and measurements of apparent
in vivo inhibition of ChE activity by such compounds as propoxur (173).
Attention is drawn also to the fact that the currently used methods
for the determination of cholinesterase activity may lead to erroneous
conclusions when applied to rapidly reversible cholinesterase inhibitors (e. g. , N-methyl- and N, N-dimethylcarbamates). In vitro kinetic
studies should be made to elucidate the nature of the reversible inhibition reaction. The results obtained in in vivo studies should be interpreted cautiously until more satisfactory methods are available.

In addition, owing to the rapid reversibility of cholinesterase inhibition in vivo, important differences in the degree of inhibition may be observed according to the route of administration, e. g. , by gavage or in the diet (174). Cholinesterase activity in the brain, as well as erythrocytes and plasma, should be measured during short- and long-term feeding studies on ChE-inhibiting pesticides (175). In this regard, a WHO Scientific Group noted that ChEs in both plasma and erythrocytes are markedly reduced by a number of substances, including many OP compounds used as pesticides. There is, however, poor correlation between the ChE levels and the signs and symptoms of toxicity. Blood ChE levels may be useful as an indication of exposure to a substance with anti-ChE activity, but not as an invariable guide to the degree of intoxication present or predicted. In general, lack of correlation between the activity of a particular enzyme, or the level of a chemical or one of its metabolites at some specific site (e. g. , in blood), and the occurrence of toxic signs of symptoms may be due to the fact that the more significant change in activity or concentration is occurring at some other site (e. g. , at nerve endings). Thus, the changes being measured may correlate with changes at the more significant site only over a small part of the range. Alternatively, some other enzyme, chemical, or metabolite may be more closely related to the toxic mechanism. Although changes in blood ChE levels may be helpful in toxicological studies, it is important that further research should be done to relate the indices used as closely as possible to the biochemical changes concerned in bringing about the toxic effects (176).

In this respect, the desirability of determining the usefulness of aliesterases inhibition and of electroencephalographic criteria for assessing the effects of the ChE-inhibiting pesticides is also emphasized (177, 178).

In effect, short-term studies with organophosphorus insecticides have demonstrated that aliesterase activity in liver and serum may be inhibited at concentrations lower than those that inhibit cholinesterase. It is not possible to assess the relevance of these observations to the determination of a no-effect level. However, it is endorsed the opinion with respect to the usefulness of determining aliesterase inhibition (179).

To permit evaluation or re-evaluation of certain OP compounds, there is a need for information from pharmacokinetic and enzyme kinetic studies, for information on the time-course of ChE inhibition in vivo, and for studies of aliesterase inhibition and of interactions with other organophosphates. Information is also needed on the influence of exposure to enzyme-inducing agents on the response to OP compounds (180).

9.4.2 Potentiation

The problem of interactions between pesticides, between pesticides and drugs and between pesticides and other environmental chemicals has been examined in detail (181, 182). It has been recognized that data from acute potentiation studies on ChE-inhibiting pesticides are of little direct value in assessing ADIs for man. However, they are of

value in assessing potential hazards to persons applying pesticides.
It has been noted that no evidence of potentiation was detected when
several acutely synergistic pairs of compounds were administered in
short-term tests on experimental animals at low dietary levels. It has
been suggested that consideration be given to the usefulness of inhibition of carboxylesterases ("aliesterases") as a criterion for assessing
a no-effect level of these compounds which inhibit carboxylesterases
at lower concentrations than those that inhibit cholinesterases. Recent
short-term feeding studies have demonstrated that a large number of
OP insecticides are more potent inhibitors of liver and serum carboxylesterases at lower concentrations than those that inhibit cholinesterases.
Recent short-term feeding studies have demonstrated that a large number of OP insecticides are more potent inhibitors of liver and serum
carboxylesterases than of cholinesterases. Although there is strong
evidence that inhibition of carboxylesterases is a factor in the potentiation of the acute toxicity of insecticides and other chemicals that depend upon these enzymes for their detoxification, the physiological
significance of carboxylesterase inhibition is still unknown (183).

9.4.3 Other Aspects

The importance of observations in man which may influence and
allow use of considerably smaller safety factors (184-187) and the
role of data from accidental poisoning have been repeatedly described.
The general principles adopted in the evaluation of metabolites may be
found in (188-190). Problems connected with the variability of composition of certain pesticides and impurities in technical grade products
which may account for toxic effects have been documental (191,191,
193). The mechanism of action of carbamate and OP compounds is described in two studies (194,195). Signs and symptoms of poisoning
diagnosis of intoxication as well as causes of death in anti-ChE poisoning may be found in two SHO Committee Reports (196,197). Therapy
of poisoning by ChE-inhibitors (198-200), methods for determining the
activity of ChEs in human blood (201,202) as well as methods for determining metabolites in urine (203) are other chapters that may be
usefully consulted.

9.5 The Use of Antibiotics as Pesticides

The current use of antibiotics in plant protection, predominantly as
fungicides or bactericides has been discussed. Such antibiotics are in
reality pesticides and should be subjected to tests similar to those
carried out on other pesticides.
However, the problem of possible induction of microbial resistance,
the phenomenon of cross-resistance in disease organisms affecting animals and man, and the possibility of sensitization in man from the use
of such antibiotics were of concern and warrant further discussion.
The methods for residue analysis of antibiotics are usually based on
bioassay and the sensitivity is low. There is need for more sensitive
methods for residue analysis of such antibiotics. Furthermore, the
agricultural and public health aspects associated with their use should

be kept under close consideration by FAO and WHO (170).

REFERENCES

1. WHO/FAO. Principles governing consumer safety in relation to pesticide residues. Report of a meeting of a WHO Expert Committee on Pesticide Residues held jointly with the FAO Panel of Experts on the use of Pesticides in Agriculture, FAO Plant Production and Protection Division Report No. PL/1961/11; Wld Hlth Org. techn. Rep. Ser., No. 240, 1962.
2. WHO/FAO. Evaluation of the toxicity of pesticide residues in food. Report of a Joint Meeting of the FAO Committee on Pesticides in Agriculture and the WHO Expert Committee on Pesticide Residues, FAO Meeting Report No. PL/1963/13; Wld Hlth Org./Food Add/23, 1964.
3. WHO/FAO. Evaluation of the toxicity of pesticide residues in food. Report of the second Joint Meeting of the FAO Committee on Pesticide Residues in Agriculture and the WHO Expert Committee on Pesticide Residues. FAO Meeting Report No. PL: 1965/10; WHO/Food Add/26.65, 1965.
4. Ref. 1, pp. 3-4.
5. Ref. 1, pp. 5-7.
6. Ref. 1, p. 9.
7. WHO/FAO. Pesticide residues in food. Report of the 1968 Joint Meeting of the FAO Working Party of Experts on Pesticide Residues and the WHO Expert Committee on Pesticide Residues, FAO Agricultural Studies, No. 78; Wld Hlth Org. Techn. Rep. Ser., No. 417, p. 7, 1969.
8. WHO/FAO. Pesticide residues in food. Report of the 1969 Joint Meeting of the FAO Working Party of Experts on Pesticide Residues and the WHO Expert Group on Pesticide Residues, FAO Agricultural Studies No. 84; Wld Hlth Org. techn. Rep. Ser., No. 458, pp. 4-5, 1970.
9. WHO/FAO. Pesticide residues in food. Report of the 1974 Joint Meeting of the FAO Working Party of Experts on Pesticide Residues and the WHO Expert Committee on Pesticide Residues, FAO Agricultural Studies No. 97; Wld Hlth Org. techn. Rep. Ser., No. 574, p. 15, 1975.
10. WHO/FAO. Pesticide residues in food. Report of the 1976 Joint Meeting of the FAO Panel of Experts on Pesticide Residues and the Environment and the WHO Expert Group on Pesticide Residues, FAO Food and Nutrition Series, No. 9; FAO Plant Production and Protection Series, No. 8; Wld Hlth Org. techn. Rep. Ser. No. 612.
11. WHO/FAO. Procedures for the testing of intentional food additives to establish their safety in use. Second report of the Joint FAO/WHO Expert Committee on Food Additives. FAO Nutrition Meetings Report Series, No. 17; Wld Hlth Org. techn. Rep. Ser., No. 144, 1958.

12. WHO/FAO. Evaluation of the carcinogenic hazards of food additives. Fifth report, FAO Nutrition Meetings Report Series, No. 29; Wld Hlth Org. techn. Rep. Ser. , No. 220, 1961.
13. WHO/FAO. Specifications for the identity and purity of food additives and their toxicological evaluation: some emulsifiers and stabilizers and certain other substances. Tenth report of the Joint FAO/WHO Expert Committee on Food Additives. FAO Nutrition Meetings Report Series, No. 43, 1967; Wld Hlth Org. techn. Rep. Ser. , No. 373, 1967.
14. WHO/FAO. Specifications for the identity and purity of food additives and their toxicological evaluation. Some flavouring substances and non-nutritive sweetening agents. Eleventh report of the Joint FAO/WHO Expert Committee on Food Additives. FAO Nutrition Meetings Report Series, No. 44, 1968; Wld Hlth Org. techn. Rep. Ser. , No. 383, 1968.
15. WHO/FAO. Toxicological evaluation of certain food additives with a review of general principles and of specifications. Seventeenth report of the Joint FAO/WHO Expert Committee on Food Additives. FAO Nutrition Meetings Report Series, No. 53; Wld Hlth Org. techn. Rep. Ser. , No. 539, 1974.
16. WHO. Procedures for investigating intentional and unintentional food additives. Report of a WHO Scientific Group, Wld Hlth Org. techn. Rep. Ser. , No. 348, 1967.
17. WHO. Assessment of the carcinogenicity and mutagenicity of chemicals. Report of a WHO Scientific Group. Wld Hlth Org. techn. Rep. Ser. , No. 546, 1974.
18. Ref. 11.
19. Ref. 12.
20. Ref. 1, pp. 8-9.
21. Ref. 1, pp. 16-17.
22. Ref. 1, p. 8.
23. Ref. 1, pp. 8-9.
24. WHO/FAO. Pesticide residues in food. Report of the 1973 Joint Meeting of the FAO Working Party of Experts on Pesticide Residues and of the WHO Expert Committee on Pesticide Residues, FAO Agricultural Studies, No. 92; Wld Hlth Org. techn. Rep. Ser. , No. 545, 1974.
25. Ref. 24, p. 9.
26. Ref. 9. pp. 809.
27. Ref. 2, pp. 809.
28. Ref. 1, p. 16.
29. Ref. 16.
30. WHO/FAO. Pesticide residues in food. Report of the 1970 Joint Meeting of the FAO Working Party of Experts on Pesticide Residues and the WHO Expert Group on Pesticide Residues. FAO Agricultural Studies, No. 87; Wld Hlth Org. techn. Rep. Ser. , No. 474, 1971.
31. WHO/FAO. Pesticide residues in food. Report. of the 1975 Joint Meeting of the FAO Working Party of Experts on Pesticide Residues and the WHO Expert Committee on Pesticide Residues. FAO Plant Production and Protection Series No. 1; Wld Hlth Org. techn. Rep. Ser. , No. 592, 1976.

144 Vettorazzi

32. Ref. 2, p. 9.
33. Ref. 2, pp. 9-10.
34. Ref. 2, pp. 9-11.
35. Ref. 9, p. 8.
36. Ref. 7, p. 16.
37. Ref. 30, p. 15.
38. WHO/FAO. Pesticide residues in food. Report of the 1971 Joint Meeting of the FAO Working Party of Experts on Pesticide Residues and the WHO Expert Committee on Pesticide Residues. FAO Agricultural Studies, No. 88; Wld Hlth Org. techn. Rep. Ser., No. 502, 1972.
39. Ref. 24, p. 9.
40. UICC. Carcinogenicity Testing, ed. Berenblum, I. International Union against Cancer (UICC) Wld Hlth Org. techn. Rep. Ser., Vol. 2, Geneva, 1969.
41. Ref. 8, pp. 4 and 14.
42. Ref. 9, p. 12.
43. WHO. Evaluation and testing of drugs for mutagenicity: principles and problems. Report of a WHO Scientific Group. Wld Hlth Org. techn. Rep. Ser., No. 482, 1971.
44. Ref. 24, pp. 15-16.
45. Ref. 9, p. 9.
46. Ref. 31, pp. 14-15.
47. Ref. 31, pp. 14-15 and 22.
48. Ref. 1, p. 9.
49. Ref. 1, p. 8.
50. Ref. 2, p. 9.
51. Ref. 30, p. 9.
52. Ref. 24, pp. 9-10.
53. Ref. 9, p. 22.
54. Ref. 31, p. 22.
55. WHO/FAO. Pesticide residues. Report of the 1967 Joint Meeting of the FAO Working Party and the WHO Expert Committee. FAO Meeting Report, No. PL: 1967/M/11; Wld Hlth Org. techn. Rep. Ser., No. 391, 1968.
56. Ref. 30, p. 8.
57. Ref. 30, pp. 15 and 20.
58. Ref. 24, pp. 13-14 and 25.
59. Ref. 30, p. 8.
60. Ref. 30, p. 20.
61. Ref. 24, pp. 13-14.
62. WHO/FAO. Pesticide residues in food. Joint report of the FAO Working Party on Pesticide Residues and the WHO Expert Committee on Pesticide Residues. FAO Agricultural Studies, No. 73; Wld Hlth Org. techn. Rep. Ser., No. 370, 1967.
63. Ref. 55, p. 18.
64. Ref. 30, p. 20.
65. Ref. 24, p. 25.
66. Ref. 31, pp. 11-13 and 22.
67. Ref. 1, pp. 10 and 16.

68. Ref. 55, pp. 37-43.
69. Ref. 55, pp. 10-11.
70. Ref. 30, p. 9.
71. Ref. 2, p. 10.
72. Ref. 31, p. 9.
73. Ref. 2, pp. 10-11.
74. Ref. 7, pp. 9-10.
75. Ref. 8, pp. 9 and 15.
76. Ref. 30, p. 20.
77. Ref. 62, p. 9.
78. Ref. 16, pp. 19-22.
79. Ref. 31, p. 9.
80. WHO/FAO. Evaluation of the toxicity of a number of antimicrobials and antioxidants. Sixth report of the Joint FAO/WHO Fxpert Committee on Food Additives. FAO Nutrition Meetings Report Series No. 31; Wld Hlth Org. techn. Rep. Ser., No. 228, 1962.
81. Ref. 1, pp. 9 and 17.
82. Ref. 2, pp. 5-7.
83. Ref. 2, p. 4.
84. Ref. 27, p. 12.
85. Ref. 24, p. 12.
86. WHO/FAO. Pesticide residues in food. Report of the 1972 Joint Meeting of the FAO Working Party of Experts on Pesticide Residues and of the WHO Expert Committee on Pesticide Residues. FAO Agricultural Studies, No. 90; Wld Hlth Org. techn. Rep. Ser., No. 525, pp. 6-7, 1973.
87. Ref. 31, p. 42.
88. Ref. 8, p. 40.
89. Ref. 24, p. 10.
90. Ref. 31, pp. 44-45.
91. Ref. 7, pp. 8 and 18.
92. Ref. 55, p. 7.
93. Ref. 8, p. 3.
94. Ref. 24, p. 16.
95. Ref. 30, p. 7.
96. Ref. 1, p. 9.
97. Ref. 8, p. 14.
98. Ref. 2, p. 9.
99. Ref. 8, p. 14.
100. Ref. 86, p. 14.
101. Ref. 9, p. 19.
102. Ref. 31, p. 10.
103. Ref. 10, pp. 9-10.
104. Ref. 10, pp. 8-9.
105. Ref. 2, p. 8.
106. Ref. 7, p. 12.
107. Ref. 8, p. 14.
108. Ref. 30, p. 7.
109. Ref. 38, p. 21.
110. Ref. 86, pp. 13-14 and 20.
111. Ref. 24, pp. 24-25.

112. Ref. 9, p. 22.
113. Ref. 7, pp. 12 and 19.
114. Ref. 8, p. 14.
115. Ref. 30, p. 20.
116. Ref. 10, p. 19.
117. Ref. 1, p. 17.
118. Ref. 2, p. 7.
119. Ref. 2, p. 11.
120. Ref. 31, p. 41.
121. H. P. M. (1973) Tagliche Aufnahme von Zusatzstoffen and Umwelt-chemiKalien durch Lebansmittel Ernahrungs-Umschau 20 Heft 1.
122. WHO/FAO. Report of Third Joint FAO/WHO Conference on Food Additives and Contaminants, WHO, Geneva, 22-26 October 1973. WHO/Food Add/74.43.
123. WHO/FAO. Evaluation of certain food additives and the contaminants mercury, lead, and cadmium. FAO Nutrition Meetings Report Series, No. 51; Wld Hlth Org. techn. Rep. Ser., No. 505, p. 28, 1972.
124. WHO. Calculation of potential intake of food additives and contamanints. Report on WHO computerized programme. FAO/WHO/C/73.5.1 (unpublished).
125. Ref. 7, pp. 19-20.
126. Ref. 8, pp. 9 and 14.
127. Ref. 30, pp. 13-14 and 20.
128, Ref. 38, pp. 19-21.
129. Ref. 24, p. 25.
130. Ref. 9, p. 22.
131. Ref. 31, p. 20.
132. Ref. 10, pp. 17-18.
133. WHO/FAO. Report of the first session of the Codex Committee on Food Additives. Appendix V, pp. 1-3. Alinorm 66/24, 1966.
134. Ref. 2, p. 5.
135. Ref. 2, pp. 5-6.
136. Ref. 55, pp. 21-27.
137. WHO/FAO. Report of the fourth session of the Codex Committee on Pesticide Residues. Appendix II: Report of the ad hoc drafting group on principles for establishing and enforcing pesticide residue tolerances. Appendix II, pp. 1-7. Alinorm 70/24, 1969.
138. Ref. 8, pp. 38-43.
139. Ref. 38, p. 21.
140. Ref. 31, pp. 39-45.
141. WHO/FAO. Report of a meeting of an ad hoc Working Group of the Codex Committee on Pesticide Residues. Alinorm 72/24, 1971.
142. WHO/FAO. Report of the sixth session of the Codex Committee on Pesticide Residues. Appendix II. Alinorm 72/24A, 1972.
143. Ref. 1, pp. 17-18.
144. Ref. 133, Appendix V, p. 5.
145. Ref. 62, pp. 11-13.
146. Ref. 55, p. 8.
147. Ref. 86, pp. 14-15.
148. Ref. 31, pp. 41-42.

149. Ref. 9, pp. 10-11.
150. Ref. 24, pp. 12-13.
151. WHO/FAO. Evaluation of the toxicity of pesticide residues in food. Report of the Second Joint Meeting of the FAO Committee on Pesticides in Agriculture and the WHO Expert Committee on Pesticide Residues. FAO Meeting Report No. PL:1965/10; WHO/Food Add/ 26.65, 1965.
152. WHO/FAO. Evaluation of the hazards to consumers resulting from the use of fumigants in the protection of food. FAO Meeting Report, No. PL:1965/10/2; WHO/Food Add/28.65, 1965.
153. Ref. 8, pp. 7-8.
154. Ref. 38, pp. 13-14.
155. Ref. 62, pp. 15-16.
156. Ref. 55, p. 18.
157. Ref. 30, p. 20.
158. Ref. 7, pp. 9 and 19.
159. Ref. 8, p. 8.
160. Ref. 8, pp. 6-7.
161. Ref. 86, p. 9.
162. Ref. 9, p. 13.
163. WHO/FAO. The use of mercury and alternative compounds as seed dressing. WHO Techn. Rep. Ser., No. 555, 1974.
164. Ref. 24, pp. 17 and 25.
165. WHO/FAO. 1969 evaluations of some pesticide residues in food. FAO/PL:1969/M/17?1; WHO/Food Add/70.38, p. 165, 1970.
166. Ref. 24, p. 17.
167. Ref. 9, pp. 13-14.
168. Ref. 123.
169. Ref. 86, pp. 9 and 20.
170. Ref. 31, pp. 15 and 22.
171. Ref. 7, p. 9.
172. Ref. 38, p. 7.
173. Ref. 24, pp. 14-15.
174. Ref. 10, p. 11.
175. Ref. 9, p. 11.
176. Ref. 62, pp. 17-18.
177. Ref. 86, p. 8.
178. Ref. 9, p. 11.
179. Ref. 10, p. 11.
180. Ref. 24, p. 14.
181. Ref. 55, pp. 37-40.
182. Ref. 30, p. 9.
183. Ref. 86, p. 8.
184. Ref. 7, p. 10.
185. Ref. 8, p. 15.
186. Ref. 30, p. 20.
187. Ref. 9, p. 9.
188. Ref. 7, p. 7.
189. Ref. 8, p. 3.
190. Ref. 24, p. 16.
191. Ref. 7, p. 7.

148 Vettorazzi

192. Ref. 8, pp. 4-5.
193. Ref. 9, p. 15.
194. WHO. Toxic hazards of pesticides to man. Twelfth report of the WHO Expert Committee on Insecticides. Wld Hlth Org. techn. Rep. Ser., No. 227, p. 8, 1962.
195. WHO. Safe use of pesticides in public health. Sixteenth report of the WHO Expert Committee on Insecticides. Wld Hlth Org. techn. Rep. Ser., No. 356, pp. 10-11, 1967.
196. Ref. 194, pp. 9-11 and 14.
197. Ref. 195, pp. 11-14.
198. Ref. 194, pp. 11-14.
199. Ref. 195, pp. 23-26 and 58-59.
200. WHO. Safe use of pesticides. Twentieth report of the WHO Expert Committee on Insecticides. Wld Hlth Org. techn. Rep. Ser., No. 513, pp. 49-50, 1973.
201. Ref. 194, pp. 14-22.
202. WHO. Chemical and biochemical methodology for the assessment of hazards of pesticides to man. Report of a WHO Scientific Group. Wld Hlth Org. techn. Rep. Ser., No. 560, pp. 15-16, 1975.
203. Ref. 194, pp. 22-23.
204. Ref. 1, p. 10.
205. Ref. 31, p. 41.
206. FAO/WHO. Pesticide residues in food. Report of the 1977 FAO/WHO Meeting of the FAO Panel of Experts on Pesticide Residues and the Environment and the WHO Expert Committee on Pesticide Residues (in publication), 1978.
207. Parke, D. V., and Gray, T. J. B., A comparative study of the enzymic and morphological changes of livers of rats fed butylated hydroxytoluene, safrole, Ponceau MX or 2-acetamidofluorene. Proceedings of the 25th Symposium of Primary Liver Tumours, Titisee, October 1977.
208. Parke, D. V., Biochemical aspects, In: Principles of Surgical Oncology, Ed. R. W. Raven, Plenum Medical Press, New York and London, pp. 113-156, 1977.
209. Parke, D. V., and Symons, A. M., The biochemical pharmacology of mucus. In: Mucus in Health and Diseases, pp. 423-441, Eds. M. Elstein and D. V. Parke. Plenum Medical Press, New York and London, 1977.
210. Ref. 30, p. 20.
211. Ref. 24, p. 25.
212. Parke, D. V., The role of the endoplasmic reticulum in carcinogenesis. Ecotoxicology and Environmental Quality. Academic Press, New York, N. Y. (In press), 1978.

GLOSSARY

This glossary contains definitions of terms (glosses) which are currently adopted by the Joint FAO/WHO Expert Committee on Food Additives and the Joint FAO/WHO Meeting on Pesticide Residues and are not necessarily of universal validity.

In drawing up these definitions reliance was placed only on the original sources where a particular term was either clearly defined or at least implied. Since definitions are end-products of an exercise of logic, no attempt was made to apply strict rational rules to terms in permanent state of fluidity such as those encountered in the jargon of international food regulatory toxicology. Thus, in several instances it was found preferable to use direct quotations from the text instead of attempting to give unsatisfactory concise descriptions of items (such as "short-/long-term toxicity studies") whose meanings have had continuous historical evolution.

Acceptable Daily Intake (ADI): The acceptable daily intake of a chemical is the daily intake which, during an entire lifetime, appears to be without appreciable risk to the health of the consumer on the basis of all the known facts at the time when a toxicological assessment is carried out. It is expressed in milligrams of the chemical per kilogram of body weight.

Explanatory note. For this purpose "without appreciable risk" is taken to mean the practical certainty that injury will not result even after a lifetime exposure to that chemical. The figure of the ADI is generally derived from feeding studies in animals and as far as possible in man. However, for ADIs related to pesticides, if the residues of a pesticide are known to consist of more than one chemical that may influence the toxicity of the residue, information on the toxicology of the residual chemicals and, when appropriate, their acceptable daily intake have to be taken into account when assessing the risk. (For further information concerning the inclusion of metabolites, see Chapter II, Section 5.4.5.) Acceptable daily intake figures are always subject to revision at any time in the light of new information (1). See also Chapter I, Section 6.4.2, and Chapter II, Section 5.4.

Acceptable Daily Intake not Specified: See discussion in Chapter I, Section 6.4.2.

Acute Toxicity Studies: See discussion in Chapter I, Section 4.6, and Chapter II, Section 3.7.

Conditional Acceptable Daily Intake: A conditional acceptable daily intake is one that is established for a pesticide in order to limit its use to those situations where no satisfactory substitutes are available (2). This definition will be the subject of further discussion (3). The allocation of conditional ADIs for intentional food additives has been superseded. See also Chapter I, Section 6.4.2, and Chapter II, Section 5.4.3.

Extraneous Residue Limit: An extraneous residue limit is, for a particular commodity the maximum toxicologically acceptable concentration of a residue unavoidably arising from sources other than the use of a pesticide directly or indirectly for the production of that commodity. The extraneous residue limit should be legally recognized.

Explanatory note. Residues in food of animal origin arising form residues in animal feed derived from activities that are controllable by farming practices are covered by this definition (4). The expressions "negligible residues" (5) and "unintentional residue" (6) which have been employed in the past, are currently superseded (7).

Food Additive: Any non-nutritive substance added intentionally to food (8), generally in small quantities, to improve its appearance, flavor, texture or storage properties (9) with the exception of substances which are added to food exclusively for their nutritive properties but including animal feed adjunts which may result in residues in human food and components of packaging materials which may find their way into human food (10), and other contaminants (11),

Explanatory note. This definition applies to the scope of the safety program WHO/FAO in the area of food additives and relates principally to the activities of the Joint FAO/WHO Expert Committee on Food Additives. Pesticide residues and radioactive contaminants of food are being dealt with in separate WHO/FAO programs and, therefore, are not included in the scope of this definition (11). However, for the purpose of the applicability of recommended testing procedures, the term "food additive" is intended to apply to substances incorporated directly into foods, those arising indirectly from migration out of food-packaging materials, those present as pesticide residues, and any other substance resulting from the intentional and unintentional incorporation into food (12). Definition of food additive and contaminant for the purpose of the Codex Alimentarius are found in the WHO/FAO Procedural Manual (13).

Further Work Required: Further work required for a food additive or pesticide is work that must be done, properly reported and made available within a specified period before acceptable daily intakes and/or maximum residue limits can be recommended or confirmed.

Explanatory note. In certain instances, although acceptable daily intakes have been established, further work has been considered to be essential to remove doubts about the toxicological significance of some experimental observations. Results of the further work required should be made available not later than the specified date, after which the compound will be re-evaluated. The re-evaluation may be done at an earlier date if relevant information become available (16).

Further Work Desirable: Further work desirable is work which, when properly reported and made available would be expected to provide additional assurance that acceptable daily intakes are adequate for the protection of the health of the consumer.

Good Agricultural Practice in the Use of Pesticides: Good agricultural practice in the use of pesticide are the officially recommended or authorized usage of pesticides under practical conditions at any stage of production, storage, transport, distribution, and processing of food and other agricultural commodities, bearing in mind the variations in requirements within and between regions and taking into account the minimum quantities necessary to achieve adequate control, the pesticide being applied in such a manner as to leave residues that are the smallest amounts practicable and that are toxicologically acceptable.

Explanatory note. The "officially recommended or authorized" usage is that which complies with the procedures, including formulation, dosage rates, frequency of application and preharvest intervals, approved by the relevant authorities (14). The definition of good agricultural practice in the use of pesticides for the purpose of the Codex Alimentarius is found in the WHO/FAO Procedure Manual (13).

Guideline Level: A guideline level is the maximum concentration of a pesticide residue that might occur after the officially recommended or authorized use of a pesticide for which no acceptable daily intake or temporary acceptable daily intake is established and that need not to be exceeded if good practices are followed. It is expressed in milligrams for the residue per kilogram of food (4, 15).

Explanatory note. A guideline level is not supported by toxicological assessment.

Intake: The amount of a substance which is taken into the body, regardless of whether or not it is absorbed.

Limit of Detection: The limit of detection of a method of analysis is the lowest concentration of a pesticide residue that can be qualitatively detected in a specified commodity (16).

Limit of Determination: The limit of determination of a method of analysis is the lowest concentration of a pesticide residue that can be quantitatively measured in the specified commodity with an acceptable degree of certainty (16).

Long-term Studies: See discussion in Chapter I, Section 4.8, and Chapter II, Section 3.9.

Maximum Residue Limit: A maximum residue limit is the maximum concentration of a pesticide residue resulting from the use of a pesticide according to good agricultural practice directly or indirectly for the production and/or protection of the commodity for which the limit is recommended. The maximum residue limit should be legally recognized. It is expressed in milligrams of the residue per kilogram of the commodity.

Explanatory note. The expression "maximum residue limit" replaces the formerly used "tolerance" in accordance with the practice recently initiated (2, 15). A definition for the purpose of the Codex Alimentarius is found in the WHO/FAO Procedure Manual (13).

No-effect Level: When applied to experimental data from animals, the term refers to the level of a substance that can be included in the diet of a group of animals without toxic effect.

Explanatory note. With certain substances the highest level that can be incorporated in a diet fails to produce any effect. However, some food additives do exert toxic effects when fed at high levels and for these the maximum no-effect level is used. The maximum no-effect level should be determined in the most appropriate species of animals and be based on the most pertinent criteria of toxicity (17). See also Chapter I, Section 6.2, and Chapter II, Section 5.2.

Objective Sample: An objective sample is a sample of a food or other agricultural commodity taken at random.

Explanatory note. The samples taken during total diet intake studies fall into this category (16).

Pesticide: A pesticide is any substance or mixture of substances intended for preventing or controlling any unwanted species of plants or animals and also includes any substances or mixture of substances intended for use as plant-growth regulator, defoliant or dessicant.

Explanatory note. The term "pesticide" includes any substance used for the control of pests during the production, storage, transport, marketing or processing of food for man or animals or which may be administered to animals for the control of insects or arachnids in or on their bodies. It does not apply to antibiotics or other chemicals administered to animals for other purposes (such as to stimulate their growth or to modify their reproductive behavior) nor does it apply to fertilizers (18). A definition for the purpose of the Codex Alimentarius is found in the WHO/FAO Procedure Manual (13). See also the definition of "Food Additive" in this glossary.

Pesticide Residue: A pesticide residue is any substance or mixture of substances in food for man or animals resulting from the use of a pesticide and includes any specified derivatives, such as degradation and conversion products, metabolites, reaction products and impurities which are considered to be of toxicological significance.

Explanatory note. The term "pesticide residue" includes residues from unknown sources (i. e. , background residues) as well as those from known uses or the chemical in question (18). The definition of "pesticide residue" is extended to include residues in animal feed and to limit the conversion products included in the definition to those considered to be of toxicological significance (7). A definition for the purpose of the Codex Alimentarius is found in the WHO/FAO Procedure Manual (13).

Potential Daily Intake: The potential daily intake of a pesticide is the theoretical intake calculated on the basis of the maximum residue limits and/or extraneous residue limits and the per caput consumption of the relevant food commodities per day (2). The same concept applies to food additive intakes. See also Chapter I, Section 6.4.6 and Chapter II, Section 7.3.

Provisional Tolerable Weekly Intake: See discussion in Chapter I,
Section 6.4.2.

Regulatory Method of Analysis: A regulatory method of analysis is a
method suitable for the determination of a pesticide residue or a food
additive level in connection with the enforcement of legislation.
    Explanatory note. For this purpose, it is often necessary to identi-
fy the nature of the residue as well as to determine its concentration.
Subject to any expression of requirements in the particular legislation,
the accuracy, precision and limit of determination of a regulatory
method need be sufficient only to demonstrate clearly whether or not
a maximum residue limit or a permissible level has been exceeded.
Usually, regulatory methods are not specified in pesticide residue
legislation, and at any given time there may be a number of methods
suitable for a particular purpose (16). The definition of "referee
methods of analysis" (19) is superseded (3).

Safety Factor: The safety factor is an arbitrary factor used in the
process of extrapolation from the maximum dietary level causing no-
effect in experimental animals to the acceptable daily intake (ADI) in
man for the purpose of establishing some margin of safety.
    Explanatory note. An arbitrary factor of 100 has been widely ac-
cepted by the Joint FAO/WHO Expert Committee on Food Additives
and by the Joint FAO/WHO Meeting on Pesticide Residues. In practice the margin of safety has varied from 10-fold to 500-fold or more,
based mainly on the scope and comprehensiveness of the data available (20). A detailed discussion of safety factors for food additives
(21) and for pesticides (22) has been published. See also Chapter I,
Section 6.3, and Chapter II, Section 5.3.

Short-term Studies: See discussion in Chapter I, Section 4.7, and
Chapter II, Section 3.8.

Special Toxicological Studies (carcinogenicity, embryotoxicity, mutagenicity, reproduction, teratogenicity, etc.): See discussion in
Chapter I, Section 4.9, and Chapter II, Sections 3.10 and 3.11.

Subjective Sample: Subjective samples include those samples taken
during the early stages of the introduction of a pesticide into practical
application, when it is desirable to ascertain the residues occurring
after known methods of application in the field, as well as those taken
in circumstances where there are reasons to suspect that good agricultural practice has not been followed. Such samples may relate to
crops from specific sites or from districts or countries where the
use of particular pesticides is known or suspected. Subjective sampling,
rather than total diet studies, is sometimes used to assess the actual
danger to consumers, particularly where the sampling and analytical
facilities are limited. It enables the facilities to be concentrated on
those categories of food intake considered to offer the greatest risk.
Subjective sampling also enables certain of the analytical difficulties
ensountered in total diet studies to be avoided (23).

Temporary Acceptable Daily Intake: A temporary acceptable daily intake is an acceptable daily intake (ADI) established for a specified, limited period.

Explanatory note. A specified period is provided to enable additional biochemical, toxicological or other data to be obtained, as may be required for establishing an acceptable daily intake (see definition of "Further Work Required" in this glossary). In such cases any recommendation will normally involve the application of a safety factor, the size of which will depend on the nature of the toxicity of the compound but which will be larger than the normally used in estimating acceptable daily intakes. In all cases the position will be reviewed not later than the first meeting following the specified date (24).

The definition of "Temporary Acceptable Daily Intake" now includes the fact that a period of validity must be specified (3).

The definition of "Tentative Negligible Daily Intake" (25) is superseded (3). See also Chapter I, Section 6.4.2, and Chapter II, Section 5.4.

Temporary Maximum Residue Limit: A temporary maximum residue limit is a maximum residue limit established for a specified, limited period.

Explanatory note. This term replaces the formerly use "Temporary Tolerance." A temporary maximum residue limit is proposed under either of the following conditions: a. When only a temporary or conditional acceptable daily intake has been established for the pesticide concerned; or b. when, although an acceptable dialy intake has been established, the residue data are inadequate for firm maximum residue limit recommendations. Residues for which data are inadequate include those for which information on losses of residue during storage, handling and preparation is inadequate and for which calculations based on the inadequate figures indicate that the potential daily intake could be exceeded. In cases of this kind temporary maximum residue limits are recommended only after information is considered on the actual occurrence of residues in food, obtained from total diet and similar studies, and after it has been shown that the acceptable daily intake is not likely to be exceeded. The information includes the results from subjective and/or objective sampling, including total diet studies, in various countries and particularly in places where pesticides are most widely be reviewed no later than the first meeting following the specified date (26).

Teratogenicity: By teratogenicity is meant a toxic effect on the embryo or fetus resulting in a congenital abnormality (27). See also Chapter I, Section 4.9.1, and Chapter II, Section 3.10.

Total Diet Study: A total diet study is a study designed to establish the pattern of pesticide residue intake by a person consuming a defined diet.

Explanatory note. To make total diet studies, random samples of food are usually purchased in representative population centers in the country or district concerned and weighed out in the proportion in which they are consumed in the total diet. The weighed portions are than washed, cooked or otherwise prepared in the normal way for table presentation and then mixed to give a number of predetermined food group samples comprising, for example, cereals, green vegetables, root crops, fruits and preserves, fats, meats and milk. These groups are chosen with the intention of minimizing the subsequent analytical problems. They also serve to identify the areas of the diet which contribute most to total residues present. The foods are purchased and prepared under expert supervision with the requirements of the studies in mind, but otherwise they resemble as far as possible the normal character of the total diet. Water and beverages are included. Each food group sample, prepared as above, is analyzed for various residues. This may involve several different analyses for each group. The exact analytical procedure may vary from group to group. In addition, from experience, it may become possible to omit certain analyses for some groups. Thus, the different groups will not necessarily be subject to exactly the same analytical procedure. Similar studies have also been described as "market basket" studies (28). See also Chapter I, Section 6.4.6, and Chapter II, Section 7.3.

Unconventional Toxicity Studies: See discussion in Chapter I, Section 4.11.

REFERENCES

1. WHO/FAO, Pesticide residues in food. Report of the 1975 Joint Meeting of the FAO Working Party of Experts on Pesticide Residues and the WHO Expert Committee on Pesticide Residues. FAO Plant Production and Protection Series, No. 1; Wld Hlth Org. techn. Rep. Ser., No. 592, p. 40, 1976.
2. Ref. 1, p. 41.
3. Ref. 1, p. 11.
4. Ref. 1, p. 42.
5. WHO/FAO, Pesticide residues in food. Report of the 1971 Joint Meeting of the FAO Working Party of Experts on Pesticides Residues and the WHO Expert Committee on Pesticide Residues. FAO Agricultural Studies, No. 88; Wld Hlth Org. techn. Rep. Ser., No. 502, p. 38, 1972.
6. Ref. 5, p. 20.
7. Ref. 1, p. 10.
8. WHO/FAO, General principles governing the use of food additives. First report of the Joint FAO/WHO Expert Committee on Food Additives. FAO Nutrition Meeting Report Series, No. 15; Wld Hlth Org. techn. Rep. Ser., No. 129, p. 3, 1957.
9. WHO/FAO, Joint FAO/WHO Expert Committee on Nutrition. Fourth report. FAO Nutrition Meetings Report Series, No. 9; Wld Hlth Org. techn. Rep. Ser., No. 97; p. 30, 1955.

10. WHO/FAO, Second Joint FAO/WHO Conference on Food Additives. FAO Nutrition Meetings Report Series, No. 34; Wld Hlth Org. techn. Rep. Ser., No. 264, p. 4, 1963.
11. WHO/FAO, Report of the Third Joint FAO/WHO Conference on Food Additives and Contaminants. FAO Miscellaneous Meetings Report Series, ESN:MMS 74/6; WHO/Food Add./74.43, p. 9, 1974.
12. WHO, Procedures for investigating intentional and unintentional food additives. Report of a WHO Scientific Group. Wld Hlth Org. techn. Rep. Ser., No. 348, p. 4, 1967.
13. WHO/FAO, Procedural Manual. Joint FAO/WHO Food Standards Programme, Codex Alimentarius Commission. Fourth Edition, p. 26, 1975.
14. Ref. 1, pp. 39-40.
15. Ref. 1, p. 11.
16. Ref. 1, p. 44.
17. WHO/FAO, Toxicological evaluation of certain food additives with a review of general principles and of specifications. Seventeenth report of the Joint FAO/WHO Expert Committee on Food Additives. FAO Nutrition Meetings Report Series, No. 53; Wld Hlth Org. techn. Rep. Ser., No. 539, p. 9, 1974.
18. Ref. 1, p. 39.
19. Ref. 5, p. 43.
20. Ref. 12, pp. 19-20.
21. Vettorazzi, G., Safety factors and their application in toxicological evaluations. In: The Evaluation of Toxicological Data for the Protection of Public Health. W. J. Hunter and J. G. P. M. Smeets, Eds. Published for the Commission of the European Communities by Pergamon Press, Oxford, pp. 207-223, 1977.
22. Vettorazzi, G., Toxicological decisions and recommendations resulting from the safety assessment of pesticide residues in food. CRC Critical Rev. Toxicol. 4, 125-183, 1975.
23. Ref. 1, p. 43.
24. Ref. 1, pp. 40-41.
25. Ref. 5, p. 40.
26. Ref. 1, pp. 41-42.
27. Ref. 12, p. 17.
28. Ref. 1, pp. 42-43.
29. Ref. 1, pp. 44-45.